Decolonizing Pathways towards Integrative Healing in Social Work

Taking a new and innovative angle on social work, this book seeks to remedy the lack of holistic perspectives currently used in Western social work practice by exploring Indigenous and other culturally diverse understandings and experiences of healing.

This book examines six core areas of healing through a holistic lens that is grounded in a decolonizing perspective. Situating integrative healing within social work education and theory, the book takes an interdisciplinary approach, drawing from social memory and historical trauma, contemplative traditions, storytelling, healing literatures, integrative health, and the traditional environmental knowledge of Indigenous Peoples.

In exploring issues of water, creative expression, movement, contemplation, animals, and the natural world in relation to social work practice, the book will appeal to all scholars, practitioners, and community members interested in decolonization and Indigenous studies.

Kris Clarke is Associate Professor at the University of Helsinki, Faculty of Social Sciences. She is a queer Irish American who has held faculty appointments at the University of Tampere, Finland, and California State University, Fresno. She has worked in the field of advocacy with migrants living with HIV in the European Union. She has also organized several social memory projects to develop dialogues between community members and students. Her research focuses on structural social work, social memory, LGBTQ+ issues in social work, and harm reduction. A portfolio of her work can be seen at www.krisclarke.net.

Michael Yellow Bird is Dean and Professor of the Faculty of Social Work at the University of Manitoba. He is a member of the MHA (Mandan, Hidatsa, and Arikara) Nation in North Dakota, USA. He has held faculty appointments at the University of British Columbia, University of Kansas, Arizona State University, Humboldt State University, and North Dakota State University. His research focuses on the effects of colonization and methods of decolonization, ancestral health, Indigenous mindfulness and contemplative practices, and the cultural significance of rez dogs. He is the author of numerous scholarly articles, book chapters, and research reports and co-editor of four books, including *Indigenous Social Work around the World: Towards Culturally Relevant Education and Practice* (Routledge, 2010).

Decolonizing Pathways towards Integrative Healing in Social Work

Kris Clarke and Michael Yellow Bird

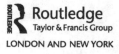
Routledge
Taylor & Francis Group

LONDON AND NEW YORK

First published 2021
by Routledge
2 Park Square, Milton Park, Abingdon, Oxon OX14 4RN

and by Routledge
52 Vanderbilt Avenue, New York, NY 10017

Routledge is an imprint of the Taylor & Francis Group, an informa business

British Library Cataloguing-in-Publication Data
A catalogue record for this book is available from the British Library

Library of Congress Cataloging-in-Publication Data
Names: Clarke, Kris, author. | Yellow Bird, Michael, author.
Title: Decolonizing pathways towards integrative healing in social work /
    Kris Clarke and Michael Yellow Bird.
Description: Milton Park, Abingdon, Oxon ; New York, NY : Routledge,
    2021. | Includes bibliographical references and index.
Identifiers: LCCN 2020018232 (print) | LCCN 2020018233 (ebook) |
    ISBN 9780415788519 (hardback) | ISBN 9781315225234 (ebook)
Subjects: LCSH: Social service. | Holistic medicine.
Classification: LCC HV40 .C6135 2021 (print) | LCC HV40 (ebook) |
    DDC 361.3/2—dc23
LC record available at https://lccn.loc.gov/2020018232
LC ebook record available at https://lccn.loc.gov/2020018233

ISBN: 978-0-415-78851-9 (hbk)
ISBN: 978-1-315-22523-4 (ebk)

Typeset in Times New Roman
by Apex CoVantage, LLC

A nation is not conquered until the hearts of its women are on the ground.

– Cheyenne Proverb

For Aune, Arundhati, Solana, Paacipiriin'U, and Hunaaneeka

Contents

Acknowledgements

Kris

The journey of writing this book has been a long process, and it has been difficult. Confronting the deep structures of colonialism instilled in me through my education and society has been disorienting and troubling, but it has also brought hope about the possibilities for a decolonized futurity through individual and collective reflection, dialogue, and the necessity of radical action to bring down the imperial structures of white supremacy.

I am grateful for this fruitful collaboration with Michael, who has been an expert, patient, and supportive guide embarking on this long path of challenging, unlearning, and relearning. I have been touched by his kindness, wisdom, and friendship throughout this process of this book. I will always cherish the memory of long conversations with Michael around a kitchen table in Fargo, North Dakota, and the warmth of his family's welcome in their loving home; thank you, Erin and the girls, for all of the genuine hospitality. My discussions with Michael have taught me so much about reimagining social work. If we do the hard work to dismantle white supremacy and settler colonialism together in respectful relationality with community, we can roll back the anthropocentric settler colonialism that continues to dominate our fragile planet. And we must.

During the writing of this book, I walked with my aunt, Betty High, through the last years of Alzheimer's disease. This precious time with her and the kind and compassionate support provided by Dr. Jeanette Rylander at the Central California VA, made me think deeply about the importance of holistic approaches when caring for our loved ones.

I will always remember the supportive conversations with Mattie B. Meyers over many years. She continually encouraged me during the early stages of this book. Her life of courageous activism remains an inspiration to me. I also want to give my heartfelt thanks to my fierce feminist sister and sharp-eyed critic, Kathryn Forbes, who pushed me through the first stages of this work and did not let me give up when the going got tough. Mike Markovich walked my dogs and was a solid and encouraging friend throughout the course of writing. Jill McCarthy was a good friend and listener during the many visits on her porch. I was fortunate to receive support to attend the Creative Nonfiction Writing Workshop at the wonderful Arts Centre in Banff, Canada, and thank the anonymous donor. I am grateful to Douglas Glover for sharing his writing wisdom. My fellow participants offered constructive criticism and support and even a taste of good scotch at the end of the course. I thank you all.

To the Donegal crew, my chosen family: John and Tina, Sandra and Ricardo, Michael and Jaime, Zoe and Holly: the laughter and joy of our time together gave wings to finishing this manuscript, and your loving friendship has meant the world to me.

I thank the many helpful people in my grandmother's town of Kildare, who taught me so much about Indigenous Irish culture. I am grateful to Mario Corrigan, Sister Phil, Kevin O'Kelly, and Joe Connelly. I will always cherish the memory of Freddy McGowan, who was always so kind to me on my visits.

Thanks to Jeannine Berger for teaching me so much by working with me and my wonder dog, Tess. Dr. Berger helped me decolonize my understanding of dogs and learn from Tess's fierceness, rather than trying to control it. I also want to thank Riikka Anna Hohti, who expanded my understanding of my fellow creatures and challenged my anthropocentric viewpoints.

I thank my wonderful and gracious hosts in Enontekiö, Anna-Maria Näkkäläjärvi, and Ellen Laubba, who taught me so much about the Sámi and their ways of life, also in relation to settler colonialism.

Participants in the decolonizing retreats that Michael and I led have brought passion and an openness for discussion that inspired me. Their wisdom taught me so much about the reality of social work and the strength of social workers who sit every day uncomplainingly and compassionately with people experiencing the worst days of their lives. Deep appreciation for Christina Alejo and Devoya Mayo of the Holistic Cultural and Education Wellness Center for making these retreats happen. Gratitude to Loren Witcher of Tools for Peace and Ari Bhōd. Many thanks to Quynh-Tram Nguyen for helping to facilitate these retreats.

A great big shout out to James Borunda, Avelina Charles, Rosa Salmeron, and all of the Fresno State students who showed true courage to talk back to power. You are my inspiration.

I am indebted to our editor, Katie Van Heest, who has helped so much in sharpening and polishing this wild manuscript. Catherine Jones at Routledge was enormously patient throughout this process.

My parents have always been so supportive throughout my life. Their love has always sustained me and I am grateful beyond words for them.

Thank you, Aune, for just being you.

Finally, I want to thank my wonderful and supportive colleagues in social work at the University of Helsinki, especially my mentor, Ilse Julkunen. It has been a real pleasure to return to Finland and land in such a thoughtful and curious academic community.

All of the mistakes in this manuscript are on Michael and me. The stories that I tell in the book are de-identified and not intended to represent any specific individual.

Michael

It was such honor and pleasure to get to know and work with Dr. Kris Clarke. Kris is an outstanding human – consciously being in the world with all of her heart, mind, and soul. She is an incredibly smart, compassionate, and hopeful person, plus a fearless and consummate decolonizer of oppressive social conditions and settler social work methodologies. She generously invited me to be a part of this writing and thinking journey. Throughout our work together, we were able to engage ourselves and one another in deep levels of soul searching and, as bell hooks would say, a fierce critical interrogation of the settler global status quo and the challenges that lay before us all.

I want to begin with a special message of love and thanks to my sons, Michael (Many Horses), Peter (Big Stone), and Matthew (A Light in the Mind). Each of you are protectors of our culture and lands. You speak out on behalf of our people, and you understand and promote the language of decolonization in your everyday lives.

I am grateful to all of the Indigenous Peoples of the world who have struggled and heroically resisted the ravages of settler colonialism which has sought to devastate their lives, cultures, waters, lands, forests, and human and cultural rights. It is no exaggeration to say that Indigenous Peoples have been singled out and regularly terrorized by settler governments, communities, and corporate interests because of their efforts to protect and maintain their way of life and territories. Throughout the world, a number of Indigenous leaders and community members continue to be assassinated, jailed, assaulted, mocked, dismissed, ignored, trivialized, beaten, murdered, and disappeared. Yet their struggles against settler colonialism are not only for themselves but also represent a larger effort to help restore dignity, respect, and the protection of all forms of life.

I thank all of the Indigenous cultural knowledge keepers around the world, who continue practicing their traditional ways so that our tribal ceremonies, stories, language, customs, beliefs, and values remain alive and relevant in these rapidly changing times. There was a time, not long ago, when Indigenous Peoples could be incarcerated for speaking their language or practicing their ceremonies. There is much that we can learn from Indigenous knowledge keepers. The knowledge and wisdom that they have shared with me have made many of the stories in this book possible.

A special acknowledgement goes to my former academic social work mentor and friend, Dr. Ronald G. Lewis (Cherokee). It was with deep sadness that I learned of his passing into the spirit world on April 16, 2019. Dr. Lewis was one of the most influential people in my life and was my social work professor and thesis and research advisor while I was in graduate school at the University of Wisconsin–Milwaukee. He is someone I've held in the highest regard; I would not have accomplished what I have today without the support and encouragement of Dr. Lewis. He believed that the social work profession, which had rightfully earned an iniquitous reputation among Indigenous Peoples because of their abduction of our children from our homes and communities, could be decolonized, indigenized, and reformed. As a social work professor, he concentrated his efforts on bringing more Indigenous People into the social work profession. He wrote grants that provided scholarship funding for students from tribal communities so that they could attend graduate school and get advanced degrees in social work. I was one of the recipients of his mental health training grant program. Dr. Lewis was, and remained throughout his life, a fierce and intelligent critic of colonialism. Through his research, academic commentary, and policy analysis, he helped to identify and conceptualize the oppressive artefacts of settler colonialism embedded in professional social work practice and then provided a roadmap of how to decolonize and indigenize social work to serve the interests of Indigenous Peoples.

One of the things I admired most about him was his identity as an Indigenous social work scholar-activist. He was at Wounded Knee (in South Dakota) during the conflict in 1973 and was at Alcatraz Island during the takeover by the American Indian Movement in 1969. He was the first American Indian to receive a PhD in social work and was named "The Father of American Indian Social Work" by the National Association of Social Workers (NASW). I was fortunate to have him as a friend, confidant, and professor and to be in his first cohort of graduate Native American social work students. I wish every person would have the blessing of someone in their academic and personal life as important as Dr. Lewis was to me. I'm sure he is now teaching in the spirit world. As Dr. Lewis often said, "Our learning never ceases."

Before and during the writing of this book, many, many close family members, relatives, and friends have passed into the spirit world. All of them died prematurely and tragically from the diseases of settler colonialism. In particular, I wish to remember Marlon Yellow Bird, Chuck Yellow Bird, Glen (Cookie) Yellow Bird, Allen (Pony) Yellow Bird, Glen (Willie) Perkins, Russell Everette, Marlon Everette, Calvin Dragswolf, Loren Lee White, Ronnie Smith, Sam Meyers, Clyde Bearstail, Bennie Hosie, Robert Grady, Cheryl Yellow Bird, Carla Yellow Bird (a missing and murdered Indigenous woman), and Janice Smith.

Introduction

The world we live in today is fraught with daunting challenges arising from a long history of the colonization and exploitation of one another and the planet. The Western values that have arisen from the legacy of colonialism have created a world of contradictions: While some enjoy a life of privilege due to their gender, skin color, sexual orientation, or income, others are embroiled in struggles that range from the pounding of daily microaggressions to life-threatening circumstances steeped in gender, sexual, and racial violence. There is no question that we are entrapped in social, political, and economic systems of our own making that undermine healthy relationships, that divide us into fearful and conflict-ridden factions, and that make us sick.

Our damaged systems are burdened by another major issue: book after book and study after study have meticulously described the environmental crises in which we are now living. Many of us are witnessing, firsthand and in real time, the increased natural and unnatural disasters that are unfolding around us. There are serious concerns as to whether human beings are willing to change their behavior to alter climate change, growing inequality, ceaseless divisions, and war. As community members and social workers, we are explicitly tasked with being agents of social change, but how can we meet these overwhelming challenges to create a more equitable world, while protecting and living in balance with Mother Earth?

It may be that the fate of humanity lies with the decisions we make from this point forward. This book invites social workers, students, and community members to imagine decolonizing pathways towards integrative social work. The relentless and invasive politics of hate, fear, racism, and neoliberalism indicate that the present social work paradigm is not equipped to engage in meaningful structural change and is in desperate need of transformation. While there are grassroots movements engaging in positive, meaningful change, the journey is challenging, and setbacks are frequent. More often than not, we are estranged from one another, from our environment, and from the sustainable practices and wisdom of our ancestors that we have not fully brought into social work practice, research, policy, and education. While we as the authors of this work hold a great deal of hope and optimism, we also accept that we live in a troubled world where optimism and solidarity appear to be in short supply, especially for the most marginalized of our sisters and brothers. Though the poet W. H. Auden already wrote in 1947 about people living in the age of anxiety, isolated and purposeless amidst material wealth, the issues facing contemporary humanity appear ever more stark and existential. We are now living in the shadows of a man-made, unnatural, mass "sixth extinction" (Kolbert, 2014). As we stand by or ignore these realities without engaging in clear solutions to reverse our course, it is little wonder that anxiety, depression, and panic disorders are among the most common psychological issues of our time.

Many people know what is happening but appear to be paralyzed and resigned to the belief that fundamentally transformative changes are not possible. This is certainly not a view to which we, as social workers, should subscribe. We must remain hopeful and engaged in social change. But a constant problem is that we in social work typically do not frame our practice as one of big, structural changes. Instead, we tend to regard tackling the big issues, such as climate crisis, institutional racism, colonialism, and predatory neoliberalism, as the duty of others. It is safer and more acceptable to work on a smaller scale, where we are rewarded by treating the current traumas of our service users, as a series of medicalized disorders managed by helping practices that are often indistinct from methods of social control. We can even thrust our clients into further distress by entangling them in colonized systems of care. To address the epidemic of disconnection, angst, fear, worry, and loss of hope, we discuss in this book how the consequences of historical trauma are intertwined with cultural repression of healing practices. We consider ways to use memory work and decolonization approaches to build pathways towards integrative healing at the individual, community, and natural environmental levels. Without any intention of cultural appropriation, we respectfully ask what sustainable beliefs and practices of Indigenous Peoples, in this present time, can help social work reconsider and reform its ways of being, knowing, and acting? How might we build truly participatory and democratic alliances between settlers and Indigenous Peoples to accomplish this task?

Social work emerged as a "modern" Western profession in step with settler colonial nation-building projects in the late nineteenth century. Its aim has been – paradoxically – to challenge state policies and advocate for social justice while supporting and operating with oppressive colonizing structures. Indeed, social work practices have sought to integrate citizens into the norms of dominant society by enforcing state policies that have routinely ignored diverse differences, needs, and experiences. Long before the US Department of Homeland Security was established in 2003 to track terrorism, treason, border security, customs, and emergencies, social workers were mandated by the state to use surveillance tools such as investigations, documentation, and case management to monitor whether individuals are eligible for benefits or services or in violation of their bureaucratically prescribed behaviors and responsibilities. Whether they want to or not and whether the rules violate the social work's core values of service, dignity, and the intrinsic worth of a human being, social workers are required to utilize professionalized techniques of boundary setting and rapport building to ensure clients' compliance (a code word for obedience, submission, and subordination).

Continually subjected to these conflicting demands, the social worker is expected to serve two masters: the state and the client. It is little wonder, then, that pervasive stress, anxiety, and burnout increasingly characterize the profession across borders. The intrinsic contradictions of the demands of expanding complex caseloads, diminishing capacities and resources, long working hours with little sense of solidarity and support, and the lack of a radical vision for social transformation in these uncertain times often feels like more than one can bear. Fighting for the interests of the most vulnerable is difficult when social work is funded and tasked by the state to implement austerity measures that hurt the well-being our communities, as the state increasingly retreats from ensuring people's basic welfare.

To understand and address the epidemics of uncertainty and angst, we are convinced that as we face the existential threat of climate crisis, we must fundamentally reimagine what social work is. We must go outside the social services industrial complex and think creatively, revisiting the older cultural and environmental philosophies and practices of our ancestors and with this knowledge mindfully challenge the oppressive structures and thinking confronting and being reproduced in social work. It may be that we no longer have to occupy small spaces with protest signs and march down the streets and ask the system for change. Social workers are part of the system, and perhaps the most successful and subversive act in creating change could be for them to be actively engaged with the decolonized practices of our ancestors. Rather than focusing efforts on trying to change the colonizers, social workers might start instead with our own transformation as individuals and as a profession. Decolonizing pathways to holistic thinking and integrative healing are often untraveled, forgotten, and avoided but are as relevant today as they were many generations ago. We also believe that if you heal the person, you can heal the planet.

In this book, our paradigm shift is the interrogation of a major scientific and philosophical heritage that underlies the discipline of social work: the idea that human beings are the most significant form of life in the universe. Anthropocentrism holds that few things in their natural state are sacred and that everything is here to be sold and profited from and exists for the benefit of humans. We are guided by Indigenous wisdom that this is not so and that if we wish to continue as a species, we must learn from the past and apply that knowledge to the present. In this spirit, we use our decolonizing lens to examine how six core practice areas – water, creative expression, movement, quiet, fellow creatures, and Mother Earth – can guide, reshape, and decolonize the present social work practice and knowledge paradigm.

Our approach is aimed at decentering the dominant settler colonial Western viewpoint by unfolding the complexity of each of the six elements that we discuss (though we recognize that there are many more that could have been included). Each chapter in this book begins with a nonfiction story that encapsulates the contradictions surrounding each core area. The stories are also meant to heal and to inspire us not to stop at healing the human but also to create practices that help to heal Mother Earth. We explore the meaning of the story through the gaps between the current state of affairs, wellness, and the dominant structures that define our action. We then discuss alternative ways of considering these core areas as healing mechanisms and provide examples to explore the possibilities of how integrative social work approaches can become useful decolonizing practices. We write this book with the hope and optimism that social work as a field can increasingly embrace diverse ways of knowing and being – that it can reconnect itself to the sacred and resist efforts to narrow our vision of what constitutes evidence and support acting in conscious social solidarity.

We do not address solely social workers with this book but seek to reach out other professionals and grassroots community leaders as well as to general readers interested in issues of social justice, collective change, and healing. Just as these complex contemporary social problems have compound, multifaceted, and deep roots resisting narrow solutions, we must also broaden discussions beyond our inner circle and familiar discourses. We make no bones about presenting our discussion of decolonizing integrative social work and healing from our own perspective. Our goals are to extend a discourse that recognizes that much is at stake for all of us and to encourage broad conversations that include those who are committed to transformation at the local and global levels.

We need our courage and action to overcome the continuous background noise of pontificating pundits, dismal economic news, mass shootings, and never-ending war. We must not become bystanders or preoccupied merely with the virtual realities of voyeurism, performing, heckling, and shaming on social media. Inaction reduces our everyday lived experience into fearful episodes of hypervigilance, torpor, and evasion. Despite social welfare systems crumbling and inequality growing, social workers can transform their profession to fulfill its mission to act in solidarity with those suffering most in society. Social work as a field can reimagine its ways of being, knowing, and acting to drive transformative environmental, social, and personal change.

We start this introduction from an Indigenous point of departure, acknowledging that we are writing this work on the lands and territories of Indigenous Peoples. Kris wrote half of this text in Fresno, California, on the traditional territories of the Yokuts, Miwok, and Mono Peoples and the other half in Finland, whose northern territories are Sámi land. Michael wrote his sections while at North Dakota State University in Fargo, North Dakota, which is located on Dakota and Anishinaabe territory, and in Winnipeg, Canada, which is located on the traditional territories of the Anishinaabe, Dakota, Oji-Cree, Cree, Dene, and Metis Peoples. We consider our acknowledgement to be an act of decolonization and a demonstration of our respect for the Indigenous custodians of these lands. We encourage readers to share this message and practice of always acknowledging the Indigenous Peoples whose territory that they (you) are visiting or occupying.

Decolonization means undoing the effects of colonization by consciously considering to what degree we and the world we live in have been manipulated, controlled, misled, and silenced by the processes and structures of colonialism. With this knowledge, we seek to engage in truth-telling, intelligent and calculated resistance, and decolonized nation-rebuilding that honors people, the stories, and the environment. We see decolonization as a critical process that challenges absences in prevailing histories, dominant anthropocentric frameworks of knowledge, governing conceptions of human diversity, and oppressive structures of managing needs and caring in society. In this book, decolonization also refers to the repatriation of what was taken from Indigenous Peoples, such as lands, waters, sacred items, their stories, their dignity, and histories. The challenge is whether social workers can be part of this legacy of justice; we believe that we can.

The path of this book

The path of this book leads us on an exploration of holistic pathways towards integrative healing: How can we in the field of social work, along with community members, imagine ways of healing ourselves and our communities and be free from the toxic legacy of settler colonialism in the current context of global neoliberalism? Can we shift social work from executing the demands of imperious bureaucratic policies to actively creating spaces of healing? Can we challenge the oppressive structures that perpetuate trauma by restoring memory and therapeutic cultural practices?

We start this book in Chapter 1 by exploring how being, knowing, and acting have been historically and deliberately constructed in Western social science to advance the canon of settler colonialism. The aim of our approach is to better understand the context of how ideas and practices of social work emerged under conditions of settler colonialism and white supremacy. We consider how the rise of various persecuting societies in Europe and the enactment of the Doctrine of Discovery combined to produce a system of settler colonialism that continues to dominate our ways of understanding ourselves and others.

We then move on in Chapter 2 to examine the impact of postcolonial trauma and the role of memory to open up the significance of speaking truth and remembering as healing acts. Postcolonial trauma continues to resonate down through the generations at a high cost to individuals and communities. By using the term "postcolonial," we do not mean to imply that colonial trauma ends and a distinct after-period begins. The trauma is continuous. We use the term to mean that the colonial trauma of genocide, removal from one's lands, and the loss of territories is translated into new kinds of trauma, such as heightened rates of alcoholism, suicide, and violence. We explore the burgeoning field of trauma studies and argue that we cannot cure symptoms without addressing the root causes of distress. We look at the progression from settler colonialism to contemporary neoliberalism to better understand the evolutionary links between the two historical moments.

The notion of professional imperialism is discussed in Chapter 3 along with Indigenous approaches to healing. We examine decolonizing social work as a means of interrogating the instruments and methods of contemporary social work practice. We explore how a decolonized and integrative social work practice rejects the diagnostic approaches to distress and illness generally taken by modern Western behavioral sciences, practices that often do not serve even the dominant and most privileged populations. Drawing on Indigenous sources, integrative approaches seek to unify the diverse aspects of the self, nature, and society to promote personal and collective healing. In exploring these issues, we want to be clear that our intention is not to appropriate or misuse Indigenous knowledge but rather to expand our professional repertoire for understanding and accessing healing practices.

The core of this book consists of six chapters that briefly examine distinct aspects of healing that are often excluded from mainstream social work interventions but which play a central role in decolonization and healing: water, creative expression, quiet and contemplation, fellow creatures, and Mother Earth. We explore these diverse elements to open up some of the critical dimensions of distress and healing that cannot be tackled piecemeal or through the narrow confines of diagnostic criteria. In exploring these elements, we consider the role of healing in relation to place, identity, physicality, mindfulness, inter-species connection, and the wholeness of our existence. We consider ways that these aspects of healing can be integrated into social work practice along with suggestions that incorporate an active resistance to the ideological and material forces of settler colonialism.

We end with a discussion of futurity, recognizing that decolonizing social work is really about radical social transformation. With the book, we aspire to open a conversation with activists, academics, social workers, and citizens of the world. Neoliberalism has become the nuclear option of settler colonialism and has commodified and monetized systems of care and help. We aim to contribute to the development of resistance to our colonized realities by encouraging new ideas and opportunities for healing as we move towards a more hopeful, participatory, and egalitarian future.

Decolonizing starting points

The history that most of us know about the modern West is a settler history; it is an unending story of exploration and settler triumph that has successfully eliminated the Indigenous voice, presence, settlement, and knowledge of lands around the world. These histories bolster settler identities and achievements but are very problematic for Indigenous Peoples. These narratives are embedded in systems of knowledge that depart from the certitude that Europeans 'discovered' a 'new world' that needed to be 'claimed,' and 'civilized.' To challenge and decolonize settler history is therefore an act of intellectual liberation that corrects a distorting chronicle of imperialist discovery and progress that has been maintained far too long by Europeans and European Americans, Canadians, Australians, and New Zealanders, among others. Thus, we open this book with a brief decolonized acknowledgment of the original peoples and cultures that have been here since time immemorial. While in this section we focus mostly on the Indigenous Peoples of the Americas, we acknowledge that similar processes and achievements have occurred around the world.

Prior to invasion and colonization by Europeans and their American descendants, tens of millions of Indigenous Peoples resided throughout the Western Hemisphere, forming hundreds of diverse groups and speaking thousands of different languages. Indigenous Peoples established individual, group, and confederated territories across the continent. They built complex networks of transcontinental trade and commerce that converged in ancient urban centers such as Cahokia, the largest city north of Mexico, which was as large as London and had a population of 10,000 people (Kehoe, 2013). Like other earthworks by the Ohio Hopewell people and Newgrange in Ireland, the people of Cahokia made constructions aligned with the lunar cycle representing complex cosmologies and astronomical capacities (Pauketat, Alt, and Kruchten, 2017). Indigenous Peoples were builders of great structures, many of them having deep spiritual significance. Indigenous-engineered pyramids, ancestral temples, and earthen mounds memorialize their interactions with animals, deities, and spiritual forces of the earth. Many of the mounds built by Indigenous Peoples in North American were effigies of serpents, panthers, and other sacred creatures and dated back from 3000 B.C.E. to 1600 C.E. (Milner, 2004).

Before the invasion of Columbus and his antecedents, the Western Hemisphere was brimming with trade and contact between different Indigenous Peoples. In what is now the United States, Canada, Mexico, and Central and South America, Indigenous Peoples created extensive trade routes. One of the more traveled and impressive is the 'Old North Trail in North America,' which stretched 2,000 miles from Canada to Mexico (Milner, 1998; Slater, Hedman, and Emerson, 2014). It is said that different tribes traveled this route to trade, marry into other tribes, and exchange ceremonies, knowledge, and culture. Indigenous Peoples have left many signs and symbols to show they were there. In North Carolina (Eastern Cherokee country), carvings on the famous Judaculla Rock, the largest example of an American Indian petroglyph, date back 3,600 years. Petroglyphs are found in the United States stretching from Alaska to the US Virgin Islands.

Indigenous Peoples weathered, survived, and adapted to drastic climate and environmental changes. The sustainability of ancient North Americans was based on their understanding of and long-term interconnectedness with the ecosystems they inhabited (Munoz, Gajewski, and Peros, 2010). In California, for example, Indigenous Peoples used prescribed burns for millennia to maintain forest health (Hankins, 2013). As conditions of drought and wildfire have grown with climate change, the US Forest Service has been increasingly interested in exploring Indigenous ways of managing forests (Lewis, 2015). For thousands of years, Indigenous Peoples have thrived by altering their behavior as drastic climate changes have occurred. Rather than fade away and die out during these periods of ecological disaster, the evidence shows that the material and agricultural cultures of Indigenous Peoples evolved to ensure their survival. Contemporary scientists are increasingly examining many of the sustainable practices of local Indigenous cultures to better understand ways of adapting to a rapidly shifting environment (Mistry and Berardi, 2016).

The archaeological and anthropological record reveals that, amongst Indigenous Peoples around the world, complex societies existed, featuring diverse social organizations spanning centralized and decentralized democracies, empires, monarchies, and inherited governance, all embedded within patriarchal, matriarchal, or shared systems of power. Many varieties of complex ideas, philosophies, technologies, mathematics, engineering, and sciences of various groups cycled through periods of zenith and nadir long before invasion. And although there was much diversity in this part of the planet, there is a clear, unmistakable symbolic and moral convergence among socially and geographically disparate peoples, indicating a broader homogeneous alliance of thought and culture.

When Europeans arrived on the American continent, they found survival difficult at best. Settlers in the early colonies would not have managed had it not been for the local Indigenous groups they encountered (Takaki, 1994). Inadequate supplies, unfamiliarity with the climate and landscapes, food shortages, and disease created starvation, illness, and high rates of mortality among the newcomers. Seeing the pitiful, destitute condition of the strangers, various Indigenous groups brought them sustenance, taught them how to survive the harsh winters, provided them with medicine, and gave them seeds for planting (Takaki, 1993). The historical record is clear: While Indigenous Peoples felt compelled to help the new colonists, they were unambiguous in stating that that the colonists should advance no farther into their territory. But, of course, colonialism and expansionism know no such limitations, nor do they respect such language.

In less than 500 years' time, European and American diseases, warfare, enslavements, and invasions had destroyed, plundered, displaced, and reduced the number of Indigenous Peoples by 50% to 90% (Dobyns and Swagerty, 1983). The complex, vibrant, and thriving Indigenous worlds progressively fell into disarray and disintegrated, some beyond repair, and some completely vanishing without a full accounting of their history and existence. Based on plenty of evidence, historian David Stannard (1992), among others, has framed the consequences of this period of the settler colonial invasion as the "American Holocaust."

During the nineteenth and twentieth centuries, groups of Indigenous Peoples found themselves deeply embroiled in heroic but unsuccessful attempts to protect their way of life, lands, and children. At the hands of American colonizers, they experienced great losses of traditional lands, waterways, and hunting and gathering territories; indeed, every treaty struck to protect the lands and territories of Indigenous Peoples was violated by the United States. During this era, they were removed, relocated, moved again, hunted down, denied occupation of their sacred sites, and finally confined, in destitution, to reservations, rancherias, and other small parcels of marginal, often uninhabitable, lands. Ceremonies that had sustained and healed them were banned, as were the languages and traditional practices that served to give them identity, connection, and well-being. In time they began to lose their tradition-keepers to disease, loneliness, starvation, and neglect. Soon they had little agency over the lives of their own children, who were taken from their villages and sent to boarding schools sometimes hundreds and hundreds of miles away. The goal of these schools was to destroy the culture of Indigenous Peoples by "killing the Indian and saving the man" (Churchill, 2004). In the boarding school environment, children were at the mercy of their new guardians, many experiencing numerous acts of racism, hate, and physical, sexual, and spiritual abuse. Often parents were prohibited from seeing their abducted children, and for some, it would be years before they would be reunited; for others, it would never happen (Adams, 1995). The kidnapping and enslavement of Indigenous children is a hallmark of settler colonial societies, and this pattern was repeated with the Sámi in Lapland, Aboriginal Australians, and First Nations in Canada.

The genocidal systems of oppression put in place by settler colonists served to subjugate the Indigenous and enslaved and forced oppressors to dehumanize themselves for the sake of the profits of extractive capitalism and privileges of racist colonial ideologies. As we discuss in the next chapter, the traditional ties of communities built around a shared commons with mutual assistance were atomized through the settler-colonial capitalist process, causing social anomie and estrangement. Alienation became the hallmark of the emerging settler-colonial extractive capitalist system in ways that have continued to dehumanize us and harm our environment.

Our stories

Decolonizing research means that we must shed the illusion that our own stories are detached from the perspective that we hold. By interrogating how we have come to be, know, and act as social work professors and researchers, we use our stories as an Indigenous methodology, situating ourselves in a web of relationality that shows the seamlessness of the life journey and ways of knowing. We take seriously what Sara Ahmed (2006, 2) has asserted: "It matters how we arrive at the places we do."

Kris

Words have long been a primary means of interacting, dreaming, and thinking for me. I was born into middle-class white privilege as the daughter of two school-teachers in Fresno, a culturally diverse, highly unequal, and socially conservative city that sprawls in the center of California. Books surrounded me from birth, and some of my most vivid early memories are of the colors and textures of the volumes that lined my father's shelves. I can still recall many of the titles of the books and even conjure up a mental image of some of the illustrations. From a young age, I spent many hours in the local library, voraciously reading everything from dog adventure books to narratives of slave uprisings to the tales of seafarers.

My family's settler colonial routes to the United States were as tradesmen, miners, and immigrants. Our family roots are in Ireland, Scotland, Denmark, and Norway, where my relatives worked as petty officials, farmers, and teachers. My Irish origins are enmeshed in the complex weave of Scottish and Viking invaders with Celtic peoples before they relocated to California in the twentieth century. My Nordic origins run deep in rural areas, where emigrants left an agrarian society transformed by growing urbanization in the late 1800s. Traversing these migrations and invasions have been intergenerational experiences of war trauma, abandonment, and crimes that shamed and exiled families propelling far-flung diasporas that separated siblings and parents. My family has benefited from the settler colonial state, which placed me in a privileged position in US society compared with people from many other groups. Though I have sought to continuously challenge the implicit bias that I have learned in American society from a young age by trying not to be silent about oppressive situations large and small, I am always learning more about the deep layers of settler colonial ideology and white privilege that shape my sense of being in the world. An important part of my personal and professional growth has been working towards becoming a conscious and active ally in solidarity with people oppressed by the settler colonial systems that have so often benefited me.

Growing up in an era when children were allowed to roam, I was expected to walk by myself or with my brother to catch the school bus. In the late 1960s and into the 1970s, the first local, fledgling attempts were made to desegregate schools in Fresno. My parents ensured that I attended largely ethnic minority schools as a youngster, which opened my eyes to how differently people lived in the impoverished San Joaquin Valley. I passed through industrial zones with rusted machinery next to rundown apartment buildings bursting with residents, down quiet streets with small Craftsman bungalows abutting tidy porches, and past grand mansions manicured by an army of gardeners laboring in the hot sun. The arid Central Valley region, with its grapes and fig orchards, ghostlike shopping malls, and multilane avenues, languorous warm summer nights and chilly winter mornings, created a tactile landscape amalgamating bucolic nature and human folly. These daily childhood journeys inculcated a lifelong recognition that how we live in places reflects the powerful forces that shape our distinct lived realities.

Catching city buses and walking through the neighborhoods of Fresno on my own gave me the freedom to linger. Consequently, I was often truant from high school while on my extended explorations. I spent hours at the downtown library, watched trials at the courthouse, and wandered through the pawn shops, lunch counters, and the fading department stores of the local Chinatown – all of the strange and pedestrian spaces housed in this mosaic-like community. Having time to think, time to walk, and time to be bored allowed me to imagine a complex and deeply layered sense of community and place. Walking is still the way that I feel most connected to places and how I heal during difficult times.

Despite my having gone to an elementary school that strongly embraced the emerging awareness of African American and Chicano history in the 1960s, there was a silence surrounding Native Americans. We were taken on field trips to visit the California missions and learned a narrative of local history as a story of white pioneers shaping a desolate wilderness into a landscape of modern industrial agriculture. Many years later, when asked whose land I was on, I realized that I did not know, and I could not name any of the local tribes despite all of my years of meandering walks through the spectrum of wealthy and working-class neighborhoods. This glaring ignorance has compelled me to learn more about how settler colonialism has infiltrated my own perspectives, my ways of seeing and working with others, as well as evaluating and understanding the world. It has also made me aware of how social memory is intimately tied to the power relations of the present and how a sense of place can be filtered through false collective memory or social amnesia.

I was raised with race and class privilege, but I had my own challenges growing up as a queer woman in a community that was deeply instilled with an ethos of fundamentalist religion and heteronormativity. I did not come from a religious family (indeed, my parents vehemently opposed institutionalized religion), but I grew up acutely aware of the social power of judgmental and moralistic beliefs. Being bullied in school and feeling excluded at various occasions because I did not fit the dominant perceptions of feminine gender expression has given me some sense of how prevailing prejudice, stigma, and oppression can stifle us and prevent us from being our own authentic selves – and how these experiences can sit with us for a lifetime. Homophobia in Fresno is not only reflected in attitudes, behaviors, and policies but has also been enacted in violent acts such as the burning of gay bars and the gay student booth on the Fresno State campus by arsonists. In 1991, the Ku Klux Klan turned up to threaten celebrants at the first Fresno Pride Parade. Since 2000, several transgender people have been murdered in seemingly random street attacks. Despite the advance of legal rights for LGBTQ+ communities, places like Fresno remain a patchwork of safe and unsafe public spaces. I grew up acutely aware of the ever-present potential of street violence directed at people like me at any time.

I came of age during the AIDS pandemic, which claimed the lives of a dozen of my friends and made me see the existential threat that the LGBTQ+ community faced not only from a virus but also from the society around us. Many of us struggled against bullying in school and made our first steps toward embodying our open and proud identities as young adults by exiling ourselves from Fresno. During this time, my mother quietly visited a fellow teacher in Fresno dying of AIDS each night in the hospital even though her colleagues shunned him and kept telling my mother that she would end up being infected because she held his hand. From my mother, I learned about resisting oppression through concrete acts of kindness and solidarity.

I attended several universities. Reed College in Portland, Oregon, with its unique humanities courses made me realize that all knowledge crosses disciplinary borders. When I spent a year at Howard University, I was involved with various community groups calling for the end to US militarism in Central America and the invasion of Grenada. It was a time of intense reading, thinking, and discussing with fellow students about the relationship between knowledge and political action. I also studied in courses that were Afrocentric, giving me my first experience of decolonized learning. During a year at University College, Cardiff, Wales, I was involved with groups that supported the miners during the strike and visited the Greenham Commons Women's Peace Camp, where I began making the connections between gender, militarism, and the environment. On a visit to Greenham Commons, I was barred from the door of the local Berkshire village pub because I looked "like a dyke" and "one of those women," which showed me how many view the confluence of political expression and diverse gender expression as dangerous. All of these experiences made real the connections between diverse approaches to knowledge and the importance of participating in political action against oppression.

When working as a bartender after college graduation and anguishing about my future, a customer gave me an advertisement for teachers from a group of international folk high schools in Northern Europe. I decided to apply and accept the first offer. I moved to Finland because I had no idea what I wanted to do, and it was the first place to answer my inquiry. Folk high schools are uniquely Nordic: They combine participatory and holistic learning with a communal working community. I arrived at Viittakivi Folk High School in Hauho, Finland, with no winter coat and a pair of tennis shoes. Viittakivi was owned by the Finnish Settlement Association and was founded in 1951 in collaboration with American Quakers after the Second World War. Dedicated to world peace and international understanding, Viittakivi hosted a number of African National Congress (ANC) and Southwest African People's Organization (SWAPO) scholarship students bound for university in Finland. The isolation and foreignness of the place brought both wonder and intense friendships. I learned about the struggle against apartheid from the deeply painful and personal stories shared by my schoolmates. As many of my African friends were heading next to the University of Tampere to study in the first English-language master's course in international relations, I decided to tag along because there was no tuition, and I had no idea of what to do next with my life. My real education in international relations came from the many hours I spent in the smoking lounge on the sixth floor of the red brick Attila Building, not the classroom. It was there that I debated for hours with my multinational classmates and learned about Amilcar Cabral, Stuart Hall, Nicos Poulantzas, Patricia Hill Collins, and Michel Foucault.

When I immigrated to Finland in 1985, I had my first experience of being a complete stranger. During this time, it was not common for Finnish people to speak English. Not knowing the language, I had to learn to be a keen observer of people to try to deduce the meaning of statements and gestures. I was largely silent for two years until I dared to venture my first words in Finnish. Finland of the 1980s was still somewhat provincial, with few foreign visitors and almost no immigrants. Finns talked of going to Europe when they visited neighboring Sweden. They lived modestly and owned few excess material items. And they rarely spoke. I learned to become comfortable with silence and to listen more carefully before reacting.

Living in Finland was the first time that I ever experienced not assuming a certain degree of privilege, though my whiteness and nationality as an American citizen certainly placed me in the category of a far more welcome outsider than most other immigrants. The police managed immigration permits, and I had my first experiences with being at the mercy of authorities to receive the right to reside and to work. Being a queer foreign woman in Finland in the 1980s meant living with a large degree of invisibility. At that time, there was a dense shroud of silence surrounding LGBTQ+ identities in Finland. Hence, I was rarely asked about my identity or family life because most people did not want to know or pry in the strongly heteronormative Finnish culture of the 1980s, an attitude that only began changing at the turn of the millennium. What being invisible in society brings is the recognition of how dominant assumptions can limit one's opportunities and possibilities to live as a full human being. It also brings the knowledge that silence can be a protective strategy to create safety in a hostile situation. From visits to the doctor to parents' night at the day care center to registering my immigration status with the police, I became acutely aware of how power, language, and institutional practices can combine to exclude.

I did not take a social work course until I was thirty-five years old. I had actively avoided them in my postgraduate studies because they seem so detached, controlling, and oriented toward bureaucratic systems. I thought that being a Finnish social worker was akin to being a paper pusher. However, having seen the central role social work played in the lives of the entire population, I became interested in entering the field as an immigrant. I thus began my postgraduate studies in social work at the University of Tampere. In keeping with the Finnish system, much of my postgraduate social work education took place through reading for book exams. The Department of Social Policy and Social Work was strongly oriented toward qualitative research, which opened up new and complex ways of conceiving social work theory and practice. We had an international seminar made up of students from Estonia, Japan, and China, in addition to Finland, which brought multicultural voices and experiences to the study of social work. As we all came from different places and experiences, the seminar atmosphere was one that encouraged deep reflection on the word and observation because there were no common assumptions about the meaning of well-being.

At the same time that I was studying for my two postgraduate social work degrees, I was also working in a European Union project called AIDS & Mobility based in the Netherlands. It sought to advocate for migrants[1] throughout the continent who were living with HIV/AIDS. In moving across borders and in meetings with various migrant organizations, I became aware of the possibilities of social work as a community capacity-building activity. I worked with people throughout the European Union who saw activism as synonymous with social work and public health. I thus became interested in developing projects that bridged the gap between the academy and migrants. I noticed that so much of the social science research produced by ethnic Finns shaped policies towards migrants. Migrants themselves, while the subjects of these immigration and integration policies, were silenced often facing complex layers of discrimination and social exclusion both from the university and societal discourse. Social workers were not always seen as natural allies by migrants because issues surrounding child protection and counseling were often entrenched in ethnocentrism and many times outright racism. Working collaboratively with fellow migrants, we wrote two of the first studies of our communities in Finland in which we explored migrants' own experiences and views on a variety of social and health interventions. A glass ceiling always seemed to shut migrants out from the university community, and therefore discussion on migrant policy issues continued during this time largely without migrant participation. These experiences opened my eyes to how academic practices tend to mirror dominant power relations and can be just as exclusionary.

The Finnish social welfare state is comprehensive in a way that is hard for people living in the United States to imagine. It touches the lives of all people who live there. Each resident has social rights to care, and there is a great deal of trust in the system; even the conservative party supports the welfare state. Yet the heavily branded Nordic welfare state is being rapidly transformed by the prevailing headwinds of global–local neoliberal socioeconomic forces and right-wing populism. These shifts have brought austerity policies and growing inequality to Finland, as well as even more blatant racism.

Finnish social work values and ethical principles are based on the concept of equality. In discussions with many Finnish social work experts, they expressed concerns that diverse practices run the risk of creating differences in equality. But equality does not mean equity, and 'best practices' can reinforce culturally and socially normative ways of seeing and being in the world. Raising a child with my partner, for example, sometimes brought challenges for a foreign and queer parent, particularly when I was trying to participate in the usual milestones of children's lives, such as parents' night at day care. The social care workers who collaborated with health care professionals to assess and provide support to young families usually ignored me and called me 'auntie.' I saw firsthand how prevailing practices can reinforce societal norms and prejudices through erasure and by withholding recognition. Invisibility goes hand in hand with everyday discrimination. My experiences have made me think about how social work sometimes comfortably embodies a professional imperialism through its emphasis on having expertise on people and their relationships because I have experienced how expertise can be used to compel adherence to oppressive practices.

I returned to the United States in 2007 to help my aging aunt as she started down the path of Alzheimer's disease and because I could not see a place for myself as an immigrant in Finnish social work education. Coming from a Finnish context into American social work was eye opening. Although I perceived a much higher degree of comfort with diversity in all of its forms in US social work education, I also observed how encroaching neoliberal risk management in the field of social work increasingly engulfs and silences critical thinking through the worship of evidence-based expertise. In the United States, there appeared to be much greater emphasis in practice on following checklists, decision trees, and scripts. For a short time, I worked as a counselor in a methadone clinic where we were regularly required to fill out a detailed questionnaire on each client's life and substance use habits. Many clients appeared exasperated because they had to keep repeating painful details of their lives with an assortment of different counselors for seemingly little purpose. We recorded the information and filed them in large binders in a locked closet. In return for sharing their stories, which were always left untouched like specimens in a jar, clients could get their methadone, which made it possible for them to function. It often felt that being a social work professional meant spending an inordinate amount of time recording various narratives in detached clinical language to bestow a treatment that did little to alleviate the cause of suffering. Writing the narratives felt more like surveillance and voyeurism than deeply engaging with people and their stories to consider different future routes. There seemed to be no time or space at work to relate to the client without a script and no tools to work with the underlying pain and trauma that led to their current situation.

My serendipitous meeting with Michael Yellow Bird came at an important time for me as I wondered how and whether I wanted to fit into the expert-driven landscape of American social work education. Returning to the United States with my interdisciplinary European social work background was a bumpy road: Many in the field viewed me as an outsider because I had not followed the American path to becoming a social work expert. My credentials and degrees were scrutinized, my competency to teach was questioned, and I struggled with what I felt was a banking system of social work education, in Paolo Freire's (2000) words. In returning to where I originally came from, I also had to think deeply about my own story, my family, my communities, the places I have been, and my identity in relation to what I cared most about in social work. The reality around me seemed layered with the weight of social memory, class warfare, oppressive ideologies, and a great deal of human pain. Yet as social workers enmeshed in complex systems, I felt we viewed the people we worked with clinically, often without considering their context. We had little to offer them beyond minimal risk management, and this was a cause of distress for many social workers.

Learning about Indigenous perspectives and decolonization through conversations and retreat work with Michael opened my eyes to broader links between the historical legacy of colonization to how we exist, think, and act as social workers. In seeking to recapture the soul of social work, which I have always felt is deeply connected with local communities in the struggle for social, environmental, and economic justice, I have begun to understand that we must recognize and relinquish the settler colonial legacy which continues to haunt us. Otherwise we will continue to seek colonized solutions for problems created by colonization. Exploring decolonization has made me think more deeply about my own prejudices that tend to center Western knowledge and my own narrow definitions of healing practices. I am grateful for the discussion and exchange of ideas with Dr. Yellow Bird, who has started me on my path of learning more about decolonization and Indigeneity (and unlearning the settler colonial bias instilled in me), especially as I have returned to Finland to take up a social work position at the University of Helsinki. This new path represents a rounding of the circle in my continuing exploration of the connection of social justice activism to the evolving field of social work.

Michael

I have always been deeply moved by the origin story of my tribal nation, the Arikara. It is a sacred narrative about respect for all things and provides us with a sense of humility regarding our place in the Great Circle of Life. In the story, we are reminded that humans do not occupy the center of all things. Instead, all life on the planet has its place in the universe; everything is sacred and must be treated respectfully. In the language of my people, to display *sakuunu* (reckless, unacceptable, and foolish behavior) towards the natural world is the action of a contrary – one who acts in a manner opposite of what is considered to be acceptable, wise, and thoughtful. Our elders say that displays of *sakuuna* towards that which is sacred will bring hardship and catastrophe.

The first words of our origin story, shared by Four Rings, an elderly and deeply respected holy man, point out the role of humans in the grand scheme of things and the sacredness of all life:

And [the Creator] blessed all the living creatures on the earth, the trees and vines and flowers and grasses, all the growing, living things upon the lap of Mother Earth which look up to the Sun; all the animals on the earth and in the waters, and the fowls of the air. He blessed all the plants and animals, and said that they are all friends of human beings, and that we should not mistreat them, but that all creatures have their place in the universe, and should be treated with respect. It was taught that the pipe should be used to offer smoke to all things which [the Creator] had blessed. And so, it has been done from ancient time through all the ages till the present time.

(Gilmore, 1924)

I am a citizen of the Sahnish (Arikara) and Hidatsa tribal nations and an enrolled member of the Three Affiliated Tribes (Mandan, Hidatsa, and Arikara). I was raised with eleven brothers and four sisters. However, my extended family comprises many relatives. My surname, Yellow Bird, comes from an ancestor who was a highly respected individual and who was deeply involved in the village, helping others and supporting and participating in sacred rituals and ceremonies. My traditional personal name, "Chief Among Many," was given to me by my grandfather, John Fox, Sr. (deceased), a military veteran and an eminent, respected elder among our people. A traditional name is not just simply given to a person; there is an order and context in which this must be done. First, the one giving the name (in this case, my grandfather) has to be a person who is wise, honest, respectful, and humble. She or he must demonstrate knowledge of and respect for our customs and culture and be acknowledged by the community as one that has both the spiritual and cultural authority to give the name. Second, the one receiving the name has to be deemed worthy and demonstrate the potential to reflect the traits of what the name means. The naming is generally done in public for the community to witness, so that they may call upon the person being named whenever help is needed.

A ritual prayer is offered in acknowledgement that all of creation is observing the ceremony, reminding the person being named and all in attendance of our relationship and duty to the natural world: "The heavenly powers above are listening. All the powers on this earth are listening, And Grandfather Stones on all the hillsides are listening. Our Mother's, this river and the ones on her banks are also listening. The Chief Above knows it. He is listening to this person who wants to carry a name. He is listening" (Parks, 1991, 37). As the name is being given and the prayers are being said, the individual giving the name uses their hands to physically press the name into the person in order for their body, mind, and spirit to always remember their responsibilities to the people, to the culture, and to all that is sacred.

I grew up on the "Fort Berthold Indian Reservation" in what is now called North Dakota in the United States. The name of our reservation has nothing to do with our tribes. Like so many of the names of American settler towns, cities, streets, rivers, and monuments in the United States, it was named after a foreigner, the Italian-born Bartholomew Berthold (1780–1831), who was involved in the exploitation of the fur trade on the upper Missouri River in the United States.

Indians and *Native Americans* are the terms most frequently used to identify Indigenous Peoples on the mainland of North, South, and Central America. However, we did not refer to ourselves as "Indians" or Native Americans or our lands as "reservations," "Fort Berthold," or "North Dakota." These names are the invention of settler colonialism, which in order to establish its legitimacy had to dispossess us of our Native identity and lands by referring to us and our territories in terms that support the principles of settler colonialism – elimination of the Native, white supremacy, and American empire building.

I was born in the mid-1950s, during the time when the US Army Corps of Engineers, with the blessing of the US Congress but in violation of the Fort Laramie Treaty of 1851, illegally confiscated and flooded over 152,000 acres of our lands to build the Garrison Dam. The theft and destruction of Indigenous People's lands has long been the hallmark of American settler colonialism. Much as with other tribal nations, the stealing of our lands devastated our tribes and left us with a legacy of loss, disruption, high rates of mortality, sickness, and cultural collapse. Throughout my years growing up on our reservation, I experienced many beautiful and happy moments with friends and relatives. However, I also witnessed high rates of alcoholism, violence, rage, trauma, and many sad, untimely deaths.

Although I have learned of the traditional ways of our people, I was not raised in a traditional village nor deeply immersed in my culture. Like many of my contemporaries, my introduction to how the world worked and our place in it was transmitted through the eyes of a white settler school system, constructed by the Bureau of Indian Affairs (BIA). The BIA is the federal agency in the US government authorized to carryout the colonial relationship between the United States and Indigenous Peoples.

Most of my memories of my BIA school years are filled with humiliation, shame, anger, and abuse, which all started very early. In 1960, shortly after I entered the first grade, my teacher viciously beat me with a large wooden ruler because I had lost my place when I was reading. This happened to me more than once and to several of my little Indigenous classmates. However, we were not the first Indigenous children to be beaten, humiliated, and tortured by the white man's education system. It happened over and over and over again to many others, from many tribes, all throughout North America.

Settler schools and racist teachers failed to destroy my passion for learning. Although my family owned very few books, I loved to look at books and could read at a very early age. When I was too young to attend school, I would wait excitedly for my older brothers and sisters to return home so I could listen to them read their books, look at the pictures, and ask them questions. I became very attached to the stories and information in the books they brought home and to read them as long as I could, I would sometimes hide them so they couldn't return them to school so soon. Before there was an open library in our community, I would check out books from the traveling bookmobile that would come to our community every two weeks during the summer. I was always the first person in line to get on the bus and the last to leave.

During the summers, it was customary for the children in our community to band together and explore the hills, valleys, river, streams, and grasslands in our part of the reservation. Our world was teeming with all varieties of life: plants, grasses, flowers, rains, winds, animals, insects, snakes, birds, flowers, stones along the river, fossils, arrowheads, horses, and rez dogs. Throughout the rez dog days of summer, we swam in the river, which was about a twelve-mile round-trip hike from our community. We would walk the distance on gravel and dirt roads, a ragged band of brothers and sisters, playing for hours along the way and at the river. The older kids would supervise the younger ones to keep them safe, while those who could swim would float out far from the shores riding on huge tree trunks that had surfaced from the bottom of our lands that had been flooded out.

When the day ended, we headed for home, choosing different byways so that we could pick wild berries and dig wild turnips and onions to eat and to quench our thirst with the cold, sweet water at a secret spring that we had discovered. As we walked along, sometimes one of the younger kids would get tired, which prompted my brother, Loren Lee White, to pick them up, put them on his back, and run ahead and drop them off a good distance from us and run back to do the same for any others who might be feeling the effects of the long day. We felt connected to our world, and at our young age, few us ever dreamed of leaving the reservation. We loved our lands, our lives, and what we knew of our culture.

However, there were times during the early part of the summer when the reservation Catholic priest would abduct us and take us to a three-week summer catechism camp, where we stayed in dorms, ate unhealthy food, and were under the watchful eyes of Catholic sisters and brothers who forced us to pray intensely for our little pagan souls so we would not go to hell. Most of the time when the priest caught us, we would be walking down the road enjoying the summer day telling stories, sharing our dreams, and looking for places to explore. When we saw him coming in his Volkswagen bus, loaded with other captured kids, we knew there was nothing we could do to escape. When we arrived at the summer camp destination, the nuns would take us to the church basement and dress us in someone's second-hand donated clothes, which were sometimes badly worn and often oversized and smelled like mothballs, except we didn't know the smell came from mothballs – we just thought because these were white peoples' clothes, this is how white people smelled. Although most of us were only grade schoolers and missed our parents, we had to learn to adapt and engage in various tactics to amuse ourselves and "spent a good deal of time trying" to subvert the white man's religion and his God by pretending to pray when we were in church, or quietly talking about our own Indigenous beliefs and telling tribal stories about the supernatural when we out of earshot of the nuns.

After several years of attending the local BIA day school, I wanted out and chose to attend a Catholic boarding high school. I have a lot of good memories of the friends that I made there and had some wonderful experiences. But what stands out most for me were the constant challenges to my Indigenous spiritual beliefs and values. More than once, the priests made it clear that the Protestants were probably going to hell and Catholics to heaven. As Native people we were assured that we were going to hell for sure if we were not Christians; but we had a better chance at paradise if we were Catholics, though we probably had to do a lot of time in Catholic purgatory (the cosmic holding cell that we would occupy following our deaths). In this place, we learned that we would have to expiate or atone and make amends for the sin of being born Indigenous and having our cultural beliefs.

When I began my undergraduate studies at the University of North Dakota in 1972, I had already read Vine Deloria, Jr.'s *Custer Died for Your Sins: An Indian Manifesto* (1969), which was an excellent critique of the failures of US federal Indian policies, treaties with American Indians that were broken by the United States, and the disruptions and interference by Christian missionaries and anthropologists in the lives of American Indians. Deloria's book helped to sharpen my critical thinking skills, enlarge my worldview, and reaffirmed the importance of speaking out and educating others about the injustices American Indians had suffered at the hands of the United States. It wasn't until I was nearing the end of my undergraduate studies that I decided to pursue a degree in social work. I had been taking social work classes and found the social work faculty in the department to approachable and supportive of my views.

After receiving my Bachelor of Social Work degree, I applied for an American Indian mental health fellowship and admission to the Master of Social Work program at the University of Wisconsin, Milwaukee. This part of my education proved to be an important validation of my activist beliefs, and it provided an understanding and support for my ugly personal experiences that I had had with racism and subjugation. Ronald G. Lewis (Cherokee) was the director of the fellowship program and the American Indian social work program at the university. Dr. Lewis was considered by many in the social work community to be a leading expert on American Indian social problems, child welfare, mental health, and culturally appropriate services. He understood the language of American colonization and the devastating impacts it had and continued to have on Native Americans.

In 1981, I graduated with my Master of Social Work degree and returned to my reservation and was hired by my tribal government to serve as our human services administrator and tribal health director. I loved being home, around people who I was familiar with. It was a joy to rediscover ceremony, connect with relatives, and attend different cultural gatherings. Working on our reservation was fulfilling but very demanding. Funding was always inadequate, the needs were always great, and the number of social and human service workers was never enough. My MSW training was helpful in some ways, but at other times, the individualistic Western mainstream helping ideologies – such as professional distance, neutral affect, serving the individual, and best interests of the child rather than the best interests of the family, group, or community, whom the child was an integral part of – deeply conflicted with the collectivist customs, beliefs, and values of our tribes. What helped most through this time were Dr. Lewis's words to me: that

I should always look to the wisdom of our ancestors to see how they solved the different challenges in their lives.

At the end of 1985, I reluctantly left my position at home and began a PhD program in social welfare at the University of Wisconsin, Madison. During those years (1986–1992), I also became deeply reengaged with my cultural traditions and systems of belief. As I returned home each summer, many of my relatives helped me to return to the sacred. Through stories, songs, and rituals, I learned a great deal about the purpose and meaning of the ceremony and how it was meant to protect us and give us guidance as we dealt with the chaos of the past and present time. I was fortunate to be present when many of our elders and spiritual leaders told heartbreaking stories of how missionaries and the state and federal governments had worked together to destroy our ceremonies and beliefs, but through the efforts of both young and old people, they were returning as had been prophesied.

In 1992, I left Madison, Wisconsin, for my first academic appointment, with the School of Social Work at the University of British Columbia, Vancouver, B.C. In this position, I learned a great deal about the language of colonization and decolonization. I began studying colonialism, postcolonialism, and decolonization movements – which were completely absent in my PhD program studies. Writers such as Franz Fanon, Aimé Césaire, Jean Paul Sartre, Albert Memmi, Joseph Conrad, Paulo Freire, and Edward Said had a profound influence on my thinking. I also learned about the consequences of colonialism and the power of resistance reading the works of many Indigenous studies, history, and social work scholars.

In the early 1990s, First Nations peoples in Canada were engaged in a cultural revitalization and spiritual healing following their long, painful experiences with Canadian colonialism. I made friends and relatives with many First Nations folks and heard story after story about the brutality of residential schools, cultural genocide, dispossession, torture, and racism. All of it was painfully and heartbreakingly familiar and traumatic to listen to, and I often felt a sense of deep sadness, shock, anger, and resentment.

In my academic career, I have held faculty appointments at five major universities (four in the United States and one in Canada), some as a social work professor and others as a professor of Tribal and Indigenous Studies. Currently, I am Dean and Professor of the Faculty of Social Work at the University of Manitoba, where I am fortunate to be engaged with my faculty, students, staff, and university community in decolonizing and Indigenizing our campus and Faculty of Social Work curriculum, policies, mission, and vision. While there is still much to be achieved in regard to justice for Indigenous Peoples in Canada, there is an open national dialogue at local, provincial, and national levels to acknowledge Canada's history of oppression and colonization of Indigenous Peoples as well as ongoing efforts to remedy that history.

Decolonizing frameworks have guided much of my scholarly analysis and activist life. Over the years, relying on cues from my many mentors, I have continued to stress the importance of activism and the need to confront and decolonize the structures of settler colonialism and empire. I continue to privilege the cultural knowledge and survival and resilience of Indigenous Peoples, and I speak out and resist settler colonialism by writing or talking back to US empire as often as I can.

Living in this world of conflict and resistance is emotionally and spiritually draining, which is why engaging in my traditional healing practices is so important to me. My healing also comes from my practice of mindfulness meditation, which I have practiced since 1975. Mindfulness practices have helped me deal with past traumatic experiences, racism, colonization, and the ongoing resistance that comes with the fight for the rights of Indigenous Peoples. I have used my knowledge of mindfulness meditation to teach my students and Indigenous Peoples from my own and other communities. To use mindfulness approaches as a tool for addressing systemic racism and colonialism, I created The Centre for Mindful Decolonization and Reconciliation (CMDR) in 2019 in our Faculty of Social Work. The goals of the CMDR are to assist Indigenous Peoples and settler allies to engage in mindful decolonization practices and strategies to heal the traumas of settler colonialism; advance truth and reconciliation between the groups; deepen cooperation to address structural oppression and social injustice; and create progressive, emancipatory ideas and actions for the sake of liberation.

In 2008, I met Professor Kris Clarke at a meeting in Burlington, Vermont. We were attending the Global Partnership for Transformative Social Work (with the Vermont Group). Through our conversations, we soon discovered we shared similar interests. Both of us spoke of the need for a social work approach that was integrative and aimed at healing rather than expert-driven and reactive. Some months later, Kris created the Integrative Healing and Decolonization Retreat Series to respond to the suffering that several of her students were experiencing and invited me to be part of the effort. We invited a number of participants to the retreat to share what had and was happening to them and to provide a forum where they could decompress, debrief, and decolonize themselves from the toxic colonialism in their lives. The gathering enabled all of us to discuss our perspectives about healing, decolonization, and community organizing and to develop strong bonds and commitments to challenge the oppressions of colonization.

I am happy that my journey has brought me to this place in my life. I feel an immense gratification from the early influences of my family and community that pushed me to do what I do, and I have high hopes that this book and the future work that I do with Kris will serve as an inspiration to Indigenous Peoples, social workers, activists, settler allies, and communities of color to continue to hold on to hope and heal through the decolonizing ideas that we put forth in this work.

Note

1 'Migrants' is often the term used in the European Union rather than the word 'immigrant,' which is far more common in nations such as the United States, Canada, and Australia. The concept of migrant reflects a more complex non-linear path to the country of residence than that of an immigrant, who intentionally makes a move from country A to country B.

References

Adams, D. 1995. *Education for Extinction: American Indians and the Boarding School Experience, 1875–1928*. Lawrence: University Press of Kansas.

Ahmed, S. 2006. *Queer Phenomenology: Orientations, Objects, Others*. Durham: Duke University Press.

Churchill, W. 2004. *Kill the Indian, Save the Man: The Genocidal Impact of American Indian Residential Schools*. San Francisco: City Lights.

Deloria, Jr. V. 1988. *Custer Died for Your Sins: An Indian Manifesto*. Norman: University of Oklahoma Press.

Dobyns, H. F., and Swagerty, W. R. 1983. *Their Number Become Thinned: Native American Population Dynamics in Eastern North America*. Knoxville: University of Tennessee Press.

Freire, P. 2000. *Pedagogy of the Oppressed*. New York: Bloomsbury.

Gilmore, M. 1924. *Gilmore Papers, Arikara Genesis and It's Teachings*. American Indian Studies Research Institute. Indiana University. Accessed June 2020 at https://aisri. indiana.edu/research/editorial/gilmore/arikara_genesis_and_its_teachings.pdf.

Hankins, D. 2013. The Effects of Indigenous Prescribed Fire on Riparian Vegetation in Central California. *Ecological Processes*, 2(1): 1–9.

Kehoe, A. 2013. Cahokia, the Great City. *OAH Magazine of History*, 27(4): 17–21.

Kolbert, E. 2014. *The Sixth Extinction: An Unnatural History*. New York: Henry Holt.

Lewis, R. 2015. Native Traditional Methods Revived to Combat California Drought, Wildfires. *Al Jazeera*. June 12, 2015.

Milner, G. 1998. *The Cahokia Chiefdom: The Archaeology of a Mississippian Society*. Smithsonian Series in Archaeological Inquiry. Washington: Smithsonian Institution Press.

Milner, G. 2004. *The Mound Builders*. London: Thames & Hudson.

Mistry, J., and Berardi, A. 2016. Bridging Indigenous and Scientific Knowledge. *Science*, 352(6291): 1274-1275.

Munoz, S. F, Gajewski, K., and Peros, M. C. 2010. Synchronous Environmental and Cultural Change in the Prehistory of the Northeastern United States. *Proceedings of the National Academy of Sciences of the United States of America*, 107(51): 22008–22013.

Parks, D. R. 1991. *The Traditional Narratives of the Arikara Indians Volume 3. Stories of Alfred Morsette: English Translations*. Lincoln, NE: University of Nebraska Press.

Pauketat, T. R., Alt, S. M., and Kruchten, J. D. 2017. The Emerald Acropolis: Elevating the Moon and Water in the Rise of Cahokia. *Antiquity*, 91(355): 207–222.

Slater, P., Hedman, K., and Emerson, T. 2014. Immigrants at the Mississippian Polity of Cahokia: Strontium Isotope Evidence for Population Movement. *Journal of Archaeological Science*, 44: 117–127.

Stannard, D. E. 1992. *American Holocaust: Columbus and the Conquest of the New World*. New York: Oxford University Press.

Takaki, R. T. 1993. *A Different Mirror: A History of Multicultural America*. Boston: Little, Brown.

Takaki, R. T. 1994. *From Different Shores: Perspectives on Race and Ethnicity in America*. New York: Oxford University Press.

1 Grounding modern social work

In the United States, the social work profession is seen as having two foremothers: Jane Addams and Mary Richmond. A Quaker deeply immersed in progressive social movements of the early twentieth century, Jane Addams was best known for founding Hull House in Chicago. Hull House was a 'settlement house,' a residential community that engaged university graduates with the urban poor through cultural and educational activities aimed at social uplift. Mary Richmond was a largely self-educated woman who started as a bookkeeper and eventually became the first female general secretary of the Baltimore-based Charity Organization Society (COS) in 1900. She focused on professionalizing the knowledge of caseworkers through the development of scientific methods. The COS was one of the first umbrella organizations that brought various groups together with the aim of making charity consistent, efficient, and preventative (Franklin, 1986, 508). The legacy of Addams and Richmond still informs how social work is conceived and implemented throughout the world.

These two women embodied distinct approaches to social work that have continued to roil the field: Addams with her community focus and Richmond with her emphasis on professionalization. Both represented many of the complexities and contradictions of a privileged and charitable approach to the structural social problems of extractive capitalism, operating in a system fully in support of white supremacy and patriarchy. Richmond sought to professionalize social work by using evidence-based methods to find and solve problems within the individual, often not taking into account the many structural systems of oppression (Jarvis, 2006). Though proclaiming appreciation for the contributions of immigrant cultures and a progressive political agenda, the settlement movement used the language of eugenics in the quest to 'civilize' newcomers by improving the education, hygiene, and orderliness of recent immigrants (Bender, 2008). Viewing assimilation as the main route to achieving acceptance by the dominant (white) American social order, settlement activities utilized an Anglo-American Christian model of social work (Schwartz, 1999). Settlement houses were also often closed to people of color. Charles Hounmenou (2012) points out that Black migrants during the Great Migration did not find Chicago settlement houses welcoming. Few donors would give to settlement charities aimed at African Americans, and whites opposed the influx of people of color to their neighborhoods.

From their earliest initiation, social programs have been framed by discourses of race, civilization, and settler colonialism (Bullard, 2015, 131). Despite the contemporary emphasis on diversity and oppression in social work education and requirements for cultural competence in social work practice, challenges remain in the way that the social welfare structures continue to be understood and operationalized through expertise that often embodies professional imperialism. Social work (discussed in the following story in the form of medical social work casework) has not always advanced or championed the values of 'outsiders' and has, in fact, continued to be locked into the colonial legacy that seeks to maintain the structures of white settler society at the expense of those that are non-white. In this respect, social work still has a long journey towards decolonizing practice and policy.

KRIS SHARES A STORY

At the turn of the millennium, a weary middle-aged woman named Yer arrived in Central California from a refugee camp in Thailand. Short and stout with strong hands, Yer wore the struggles of her life on her face. She had grown up in the midst of a US-launched imperialist war against the people of Vietnam in the mountainous regions of North Vietnam and Laos, the native land of her Hmong people. During the Vietnam War, Hmong society was completely disrupted as thousands were killed while the region became one of the most heavily bombed areas in history. The Hmong were military allies of the United States and lost 20% of the male population in combat (Vang, 1979). After the war, the Americans retreated, and the Hmong were persecuted by the Communist victors: Villages were destroyed, and people took great risks to secretly cross the dangerous Mekong River at night, escaping to huge, overcrowded refugee camps in search of safety. Yer had faced all of the travails of living through war and then fleeing the aftermath of destruction, survived the process of becoming a refugee, and relocated to Central California, blown by the winds of war from one part of the globe to another.

Living in California, far from everything she knew and held dear, Yer felt terribly lonely and restless. The climate was different, her home was surrounded by a sea of asphalt, and she could not see the stars at night amidst all of the flickering streetlights and police helicopters. Her husband had died in the refugee camp before their family of six children was granted permission to come to the United States. Yer did not understand the language or ways of her new land. Managing bills and navigating bureaucracy were left to the eldest children, who at a young age became students of the maze of American social institutions. She spent most of her time in the small apartment with her family sharing cooking and cleaning but lost in the memories of home, both good and bad. The children quickly adapted to the foreign culture and spent a good deal of time away from home with their newfound neighborhood friends who represented the diversity of the impoverished Central Valley. Yer felt that her soul had not followed her on the long, painful journey to the new country, and she felt bereft of all support, especially when night fell on her restless neighborhood and her memories welled deep in her chest.

Soon after Yer was settled, during a routine exam, local health officials discovered that she had multidrug-resistant tuberculosis (TB) which required a long course of oral antibiotic treatment. The disease is highly contagious, and officials wanted to ensure that she would comply with taking all of the medication so that she would not infect others. The health department used directly observed therapy (DOT), a strategy common in disadvantaged communities, in which a caseworker supervises the patient to ensure that she completes the full course of medication. The aim of DOT is to identify factors that prevent patients from completing their courses of treatment and to provide support for compliance that is context-sensitive and patient-centered. By addressing cultural, financial, social, and physical barriers, DOT improves access to treatment. However, for DOT to be successful, culturally appropriate health and social workers capable of partnering with vulnerable patients are key.

Yer believed that the cause of her illness was that her soul was still lost in her homeland and did not accompany her to the new, inscrutable country. In the animist Hmong belief system, human beings have several souls, which are a source of strength and spiritual energy. If a person is separated from one of her souls, she runs the risk of becoming ill, growing depressed, or dying. "Soul calling" is a ceremony performed by Hmong shamans to reunite souls with their person, thus restoring spiritual integrity. Before embarking on the DOT medical regimen, Yer wanted to hold a soul-calling ceremony, which she believed would heal her. Public health officials and social workers, unfamiliar with the Hmong community, were unsure what to do because their mandate was simply to ensure she take the medication.

A few years earlier, there had been a similar case. In that instance, a slight Laotian woman in her forties named Sunya was diagnosed with a multidrug-resistant form of TB. Sunya had been in the United States for a few years, but her family was spread out across the country. She had found it difficult to find work and, separated from her husband, had to rely on welfare benefits to get by. Sunya was given several medications to treat her TB, but the side effects were not properly explained to her, and she soon stopped treatment because she felt that the medication made her ill. There was an occasional interpreter with the caseworker, but his ability to interpret in Lao had never been tested, and young family members often ended up having to translate the physician's instructions to Sunya. A sense of distrust began to form between the health officials, caseworkers, and Sunya as her TB worsened. She began to avoid the caseworkers and hid from them with various family members.

Eventually, the health department labeled Sunya noncompliant and deemed her a risk to public health. The health department placed her in jail as a means to ensure her compliance with the medical regimen. Realizing that Sunya came from a culture in which many family members often lived closely together, health officials thought that they were being proactive to prevent others from being infected. For many months, Sunya was remanded to a small cell with no furniture, just a bed and toilet. She was housed with people who had serious mental and physical illnesses. She lost weight due to the unfamiliar food, and she was attacked by a fellow inmate. Sunya told the indifferent authorities that she was suicidal and suffered from the side effects of the strong medications, but her pleas fell on deaf ears. There was no interpreter in the jail to explain her rights or why she was incarcerated. Sunya's family also did not understand the reasons she was in jail and sought help from other community members and social workers to advocate for her release. The head public health physician wanted to detain her for two years, until the full course of her treatment was completed, so that the safety of the public could be ensured.

Sunya's family finally managed to retain an attorney from a legal assistance group that challenged the detention order of the public health department. The attorney discovered that health officials had routinely detained people of color for TB treatment, though the length of Sunya's stay at the county jail was certainly exceptional. The health department requested incarceration when there were fears that DOT would not be successful. After a lengthy court case, the county was ordered to pay over one million dollars in compensation to Sunya for unlawful incarceration, as well as emotional and physical distress. After the suit was settled, Sunya's family chanted prayers outside the county jail together with a shaman, who performed a soul-calling ceremony to heal Sunya of the trauma she had endured.

When Yer's case came up some years after Sunya, the health department paused to consider how to respond. While their heavy-handed approach to Sunya's TB had achieved the goal of ensuring she took her medication, it also resulted in a great deal of personal distress for her and a large financial settlement from the county.

Yer told public health officials that she wanted a soul-calling ceremony before starting any medical treatment because she believed that the cause of her illness was the separation of her soul from her physical body. By reuniting her soul and body, Yer felt that she could heal. A soul-calling ceremony generally costs approximately 400 dollars for the shaman's honorarium and other necessary items. Public health officials recognized that forcing DOT on patients without their full understanding and cooperation was futile, and forced detention was punitive, traumatic, illegal, and costly. Yet they could not think of alternative ways to ensure medication was taken. Officials tried to find a way to pay for the shamanic ceremony, but the county budget would not allow for such expenses. There were no line items in the budget for culturally appropriate services nor were there discretionary funds for frontline workers to pay for such activities. Only a certain range of medical interventions could be supported by the system. At a meeting on Yer's case, the attending physician felt frustrated by the lack of options. She threw 200 dollars on the table, with social workers and nurses each ponying up twenty-five dollars until the total sum of 400 dollars was reached. With these funds, they were able to arrange a soul-calling ceremony for Yer so she could feel whole in her new country and be ready to embrace the treatment offered through DOT. Shortly after the ceremony, Yer agreed to take all of the medications and was successfully treated for multidrug-resistant TB.

Lessons on pathways

Many contradictions lie at the heart of human service interventions. These women had complex sociopolitical and transnational migration and personal histories, yet they were reduced to cases of noncompliant patients that needed to be isolated from the community and managed through force. State institutions remain largely guided by many of the white supremacist aspects of settler colonial processes of being, knowing, and acting, despite the rhetoric of empowerment and respect for cultural diversity. In the story, the social and health care system was only geared toward controlling individual behavior, largely devoid of context – in this case, the culture, history, and trauma of diaspora and being a war refugee. When Sunya did not follow the medical protocol, she was detained. Officials initially did not seek to understand the context of her reasoning for not following the treatment plan. Rather, their focus was solely on ensuring she took the medication to treat the infection. Years later, officials recognized that detention was a detrimental way to act, not only due to the sting of an expensive lawsuit but also because it ultimately harmed Sunya.

A key principle of settler colonialism is that settlers forge a new identity and system after they have invaded and replaced the population of Indigenous Peoples. People who migrate to this new society are expected to leave all of their 'foreign' trappings and culture behind to support the growth of the empire, both ideologically and materially. In Yer's case, although the public health and social work team came to understand that she needed a more holistic and culturally congruent approach to managing her illness, they were nonetheless restricted by the limitations of narrow definitions of treatment to provide care and support in any way other than compulsory compliance with the medication regimen. It was only by breaking the rules of settler society that the team could work with the patient rather than work on the patient.

Many of us go into the human services because we want to join in solidarity with vulnerable people and work toward a more equitable and just society. We may have had positive experiences with social workers who helped us, our families, or our communities, and we want to be a similar catalyst for support. But why is it that our systems of care and professional practices often force us to act in ways that we know do not support the best interests of community members or individuals? How can it be that the logic of the system and our evidence-based interventions may even exacerbate problems, human suffering, and costs? Who are we, as human services experts, really helping, and who are we hurting? Are there other ways to think about healing the individual and the community? Have we social workers become so enamored of the rhetoric of helping in social work that we do not see that our interventions are many times complicit with settler colonial state power rather than truly empowering the people (Margolin, 1997)?

This chapter considers how the self, knowing, and acting – in the contemporary Western sense – have transformed historically. Through this framework, we ponder the relationship between the development of social work and the historical, ideological, and material bases of settler colonialism that have undergirded and shaped social policies, practices, and care systems. How did social work come into being, what is its knowledge base, and how does it practice? We ask: How have contemporary welfare societies emerged from their settler colonial origins of Indigenous genocide, African slavery, and industrial capitalist exploitation to construct complicated and sometimes inflexible systems to support human well-being? To understand where we have arrived in the human services, we must examine the road traveled to get here and how it has fundamentally altered our understanding of ourselves and others and our interactions with our communities and environment.

Whether we approach social work from the perspective of Jane Addams's settlement movement or Mary Richmond's social diagnosis, we must consider how our collective ways of conceiving the good life and a just society have roots in the complex legacies of settler colonialism. These legacies include particular understandings of being, knowing, and acting that shape our ideas about distress and support, which in turn define the models that specify appropriate social work practices. Though social work explicitly calls for challenging oppression and inequality in its foundational mission, it often perceives these issues through the imperial professional lens of settler colonialism, white supremacy, and white privilege. We therefore are often constrained in our thinking and experience through socialization, education, and social structures to privilege colonizing perspectives, creating treacherous cycles of cognitive dissonance, and doing harm to ourselves and others, as we saw in Sunya's story.

Being

The sense of our own subjectivity – who we are in the world – forms the basis of how we know and act. We are animated by our inner lives and emotions, which give meaning to our interactions with others and purpose to what we do. Our inner lives and emotions are the products of long evolutionary processes, wherein culture and genetics coevolved to create unique groups, tribes, societies, and individuals. Thus, while our inner lives may be constituted by similar strands of evolution, our unique development is shaped by many critical differences between peoples and their cultures and historical experiences. Our sense of ourselves is also shaped by the social order in which we live because we often see ourselves as freely submitting to (or resisting) the prevailing arrangement of social relations and structures (Althusser, 2016, 123). Yet the understanding and imposition of the social order within and between different socio-cultural groups can vary widely. A social order can enforce a sense of inferiority or unworthiness on some members through unequal power relations while exalting others. This is why internalized colonialism can be seen as a byproduct of the settler colonial state. Our sense of being is constituted through our worldviews, language, culture, and perceptions and thus emerges from complex sets of collective relationships to one another and the social, environmental, spiritual, and material worlds.

In this section, we unpack how Western subjectivity developed historically as consciousness, personhood, and agency of being in a world that is shaped by the prevailing social order. Here we outline how the shift from premodern to modern Europe with the rise of extractive capitalism and colonialism decisively altered Europeans' understanding of themselves and their environment. We examine how this emerging sense of subjectivity formed the basis for settler colonial knowing and acting, which were exported to the rest of the world.

Premodern European societies had deep roots in the complex and multicultural ancient world. Far from being homogenous states, ancient societies were quite permeable in terms of shared cultural, material, and social influences (López-Ruiz, 2010). Modern-day Lebanon, Palestine, Syria, Italy, Egypt, Greece, Iran, Iraq, and other neighboring countries were densely intertwined culturally, linguistically, and economically. Before the early modern period, there were also diverse groups of people living throughout Europe with complex cosmologies of the world, a variety of matrilineal social arrangements, egalitarian partnerships with animals, and ways of living sustainably with the environment. As nomadic Indo-European peoples such as the Celts, Vikings, and Teutons migrated, they violently seized land and created new societies and cultures that clashed with and were eventually subsumed into various empires (Percovich, 2004). The 'whitening' of Europe arose in the sixteenth century by denying recognition of Europe's deep relationship with the immense cultural diversity of the region (Rodriguez, 2011).

Early modern Europe was steeped in the worldviews and everyday practices of pre-Christian groups that lived in harmony with the environment. In these societies, one's own subjectivity was interwoven with the natural world on which early peoples were dependent. Further, as everyone needed the social collective to survive, people recognized their fundamental interconnection with one another, however distinct their social status might be. Historian Yuval Harari, the author of several popular books, including *Sapiens: A Brief History of Humankind* (2015), concludes that a capacity for flexible cooperation made humans a viable species on the planet.

Though there were certainly many conflicts and battles between different groups of people with diverse leadership, often in competition for access to resources, the individual was not valued above the group precisely because the experience of interdependence produced a subjectivity more collectivist in nature. Christianity spread throughout Europe both by the sword and through monastic communities that provided sustenance for local communities. Irish monasticism, for example, was an extremely cohesive religious structure firmly rooted in local culture that culminated in the Golden Age of Irish scholarship and art. Unlike Continental orders that placed emphasis on bureaucratic and hierarchical structures, Irish monasticism embraced a more communitarian and holistic approach to spirituality (McGrath, 2002). Similar to the Norse peoples, the Celts had a cosmology that saw the intrinsic connections between spiritual and terrestrial worlds of existence and supernatural beings through cauldrons, wells, and whirlpools (O'Donnell, 2015, 238). For many Irish, holy wells, for example, remain places of contemplation and prayer despite the continually evolving Christian understandings of these sites.

Regional agrarian European cultures began to transform into more complex national entities in the Middle Ages. Monarchies were established and considered by subjects to be ordained by a God to be feared. Clerics advanced the Great Chain of Being, a divinely decreed social order in which every person was linked and defined by the various social hierarchies, including the roles of men and women, rich and poor, lord and peasant, the powerful and powerless. The social structures and the laws of nature were viewed as largely inscrutable and explained by the mysterious will of God, which could only be challenged at the risk of heresy, as Galileo discovered (Howe, 1994). This vertical, compartmentalized, and punitive view of God represented a dramatic shift from the circular, interwoven, and nature-centered view of spirituality in pre-Christian societies.

R. I. Moore (2009) has argued that in the Middle Ages, Europe became (and remains) a 'persecuting society.' Moore (2009, 5) states that in medieval Europe, "deliberate and socially sanctioned violence began to be directed through established governmental, judicial, and social institutions, against groups of people defined by general characteristics such as race, religion, or way of life; and that membership of such groups in itself came to be regarded as justifying these attacks." Ruling elites promoted the persecution of those viewed as 'the Other' as a means of consolidating power in societies increasingly based on a money economy with a growing gap between rich and poor. Persecution, according to Moore, became a means to suppress dissent and legitimate authority. The growth of the persecuting society thus reflected a fundamental shift from a subjectivity rooted in collectivity to one based on the oppression of others (e.g., heretics, Jews, lepers, witches). The ruling elite was seen as divinely appointed and defined by church-sanctioned social norms. Some studies suggest that how we view God has an impact on how we view others (e.g., Froese and Bader, 2008). When God is viewed as distant, retributive, and critical in a religious community, then adherents may become more fearful and less trusting and open than those who believe in an all-loving and inclusive God (Mencken, Bader, and Embry, 2009). As help and care in early modern European society were organized largely by the church as charity, clergy were the guardians of society who policed the boundaries of right and wrong, deserving and undeserving, good and evil.

The modern age in Europe was initiated by both material developments and the collective leap of imagination that created nations (Anderson, 2006). From disparate tribes and groups of people, new identities and ways of being in the world emerged as the forces driving capitalism became consolidated through nation-building. A new sense of nationalism emerged during the French Revolution of 1789, even though more than half of the people living in the country did not speak standard French. People united around a new sense of French nationalism and identity, which became enshrined in schools, bureaucracies, militaries, money, and a collective emotional imaginary that defined the essential qualities of a unique Frenchness (Berenson, Duclert, and Prochasson, 2011). Notions of the nation and belonging were inextricably linked with extractive capitalist expansion and settler colonialism through imperial narratives of pure and homogenous origins.

The age of settler colonial domination had roots in the invention of new technologies such as shipbuilding and cartography in the sixteenth century, which gave Europeans dominance over the seas, firearms, and artillery, thus enhancing their military power. As European states competed with one another, the economic system of mercantilism developed to protect home economies by building up the power of one's own state by controlling trade while weakening rival states. Tensions within European societies grew as merchants sought to have greater influence in governing as inequality and conflict increased, while the Scientific Revolution challenged superstition and social hierarchies based on divine right. The Enlightenment and the French Revolution marked the birth of a new era in the eighteenth century, which brought enfranchisement (for white men of property), social mobility (for those with access to means), the rise of the paradigm of scientific inquiry, and the dawn of settler colonialism, which thrust Europe into the modern era. The nineteenth-century global economy was shaped by the dual processes of the growing concentration of capital and wealth in European metropoles and the extensive and ever-tightening grip of settler colonial empire throughout the world.

All of these historical shifts brought great changes to historically constituted European subjectivity. Unlike many Eastern societies, in which understanding subjectivity as individuality – the sense of "I for myself" – was considered to be a negative state of being, Western societies reified the concept of the self as self-reliance (Park, 2013). As modern industrial capitalism rapidly expanded along with settler colonialism, European subjectivity dramatically shifted: People no longer constructed themselves as one with nature but rather saw nature as an external force to dominate in the pursuit of individual gain (Cooper and Stoler, 1997). While nineteenth-century Romantic poets such as Wordsworth and Shelly wrote of the profound regret for the loss of the connection with nature and the rural life, the upheaval of industrialization had fundamentally altered much of the landscape of many Western countries. Competition rather than cooperation became valorized. Economic growth and continuous expansion became the measures of societal health. Progress was viewed as an inevitable linear process that ground its way forward through ancient forests by altering and polluting waterways and plowing under grasslands for croplands.

In the modern era, the oppressive dynamic of the persecuting society became increasingly cosmopolitan in creating ideologies to justify the exponential growth of the settler colonial machine across the globe. The Age of Discovery gave birth to a modern world system based on the brutal seizure of land, genocide of native peoples, enslavement of Africans, vicious exploitation of workers, and appropriation of resources in the name of civilization. An imperial Enlightenment narrative was constructed that placed a monocultural vision of ancient Greece and Rome as the originators of Western civilization, constructing a European subjectivity steeped in a sense of homogeneity and exclusivity. A fundamentally distinct relationship emerged between the European traders, settlers, and administrators who subordinated and enslaved the colonized and dispossessed not only through ruthless force but also through ideologies of race, gender, sexuality, ability, and class.

A contradiction lay at the heart of modern European subjectivity: It embodied the possibilities, capacities, and values of liberal humanism together with the cruelty, blindness, and savagery of settler colonial domination. Many of the Christian religious institutions that blessed and participated in the genocide of Indigenous Peoples – such as the Roman Catholic Church, whose priest Junipero Serra led a brutal missionary movement in eighteenth-century California – were also complicit with the persecution of the Jews in Hitler's Germany. However, when the scale of the Nazi Holocaust was revealed after the war, there was a greater sense of ecumenical responsibility, culminating in a 1998 formal repentance for Catholic inaction during the Nazi genocide. There have been no moves towards asking for forgiveness for supporting Indigenous genocide by the Church. On the contrary, the Catholic Church canonized Father Serra in 2015, raising questions of whether the Church truly recognizes its role in the barbaric history of mistreatment of Native Americans.

With the centers of European empires in ruins in the mid-twentieth century after two world wars and a global flu pandemic, a renewed sense of commonality and citizenship infused many Western countries. This led to the construction of social welfare states that supported health, education, and well-being, securing many of the basic human rights for citizens, bringing greater prosperity, and narrowing class differences through policies such as the GI Bill and national health services (Trattner, 1998). Despite these advances, racial, gendered, ableist, and heteronormative systemic exclusions remained.

After World War II, over three dozen countries achieved independence in Asia and Africa from their colonial masters. Although colonial rule fell, relations of economic and ideological dominance over newly independent countries continued. Those thrust into the colonial diaspora – Indigenous Peoples, the formerly enslaved, and other socially excluded people living in the heart of the former empire – remained marginalized and under attack from policies and practices that sought to maintain oppressive colonial relations in fresh forms. Newly independent countries became an important voice for decolonization in the United Nations through the nonaligned movement during the Cold War. Some Third World political leaders sought to develop greater autonomy through modernizing their societies by mimicking the West and rejecting traditional elements of their cultures (Schech and Haggis, 2002). Others, such as Patrice Lumumba and Kwame Nkrumah, followed the explicitly anticolonial view of psychiatrist Frantz Fanon, who argued that liberation comes through revolution rather than reform. In his classic *The Wretched of the Earth*, Fanon (1963, 61) states that colonialism is "not a thinking machine, nor a body endowed with reasoning faculties. It is violence in its natural state, and it will only yield when confronted with greater violence." The tension between the tactics of reform versus revolution has remained at the heart of debates over anticolonial resistance and reverberated throughout social work history.

The paradoxes of the post–World War II era gave rise to the notion of the postcolonial, which focused on the complex hybrid legacies and lived experiences of peoples displaced by colonialism, and critiquing colonial relations of power. Postcolonial scholar Gayatri Spivak (2010) cautioned against romanticizing precolonial cultures and said that the task of postcolonialism is to understand the complexity of worlds beyond their relationship to colonialism. The rise of heterogenous postcolonial identities led to demands for the recognition of full personhood and rights to equal citizenship both on the national and global levels. From the African American civil rights movement, which demanded equality under the law, to the assertion of nationalism in Northern Ireland to the emergence of a nonaligned bloc of newly independent nations, those long considered outsiders began to challenge the unnatural hierarchies of settler colonial societies that produced marginalized and vulnerable populations, demanding equal inclusion in society. Notions of Western subjectivity as binary, homogenous, and universal began to fragment.

Postcolonial demands for the recognition and inclusion of diverse social identities have had an impact on postwar social welfare systems and practices by challenging Western assumptions about universal subjectivity. Feminist theorists such as Nancy Fraser questioned the notion of the fully autonomous individual (e.g., Fraser, 2013). African American civil rights activists brought their experience of resistance struggle to social work (Bell, 2014). Many social work practices based on state policies of controlling and surveilling stigmatized identities, such as living in non-nuclear family structures or poverty, were increasingly interrogated pushing human services institutions to develop methodologies in the late twentieth century such as cultural competence in the attempt to manage diverse subjectivities.

The emergence of neoliberalism in the late twentieth century as an ideology, hegemonic discourse, and form of governance produced a new subjectivity distinct from previous historical iterations of the self. Following the principles of libertarian thinkers such as Ayn Rand and Friedrich Hayek rather than interventionist economist John Maynard Keynes, neoliberals saw subjective freedom as ending state regulation, which they considered to imprison people rather than liberating them from want and potential harm. As critical psychology researchers have noted,

> Neoliberalism attempts to redefine being human, offering a new subjecthood. Neoliberalism not only reproduces the individualistic subject of Early Modernism and the Enlightenment but also refashions the individual subject: The neoliberal subject is increasingly construed as a free, autonomous, individualized, self-regulating actor understood as a source of capital; as human capital. Furthermore, this neoliberal subject is not merely pursuing self-interest but becomes an entrepreneur of herself.
>
> (Türken, Nafstad, Blakar, and Roen, 2016, 34)

Privileging consumption, self-help, and the market, neoliberalism veers far from the solidarity of the social welfare state. The rhetoric of the neoliberal state seeks to activate social welfare customers so that they become responsible themselves for overcoming travails to compete in the marketplace of the good life, at the same time that the policies of the neoliberal state militate against the very idea of a common good.

Since the turn of the millennium, neoliberalism has driven economic policies of austerity that have crippled many of the comprehensive social welfare services universally provided in many Western counties. The burden for achievement has increasingly been placed on the individual and less on the collective support of social structures such as schools, health care, and unionized employment. In many senses, the twenty-first century has paradoxically brought a radically disconnected and reconnected subjectivity as nation-states have seen a resurgence of solidarity through populist nationalism and local political organizing precisely as comprehensive social citizenship in a liberal democracy and economic security has vanished.

Western subjectivity has thus shifted from the collectivist and subsistence orientation of the premodern era to the settler colonialism of the modern and then to the globalized fragmentation of the postcolonial. Each of these eras has produced distinct subjectivities that have oriented us in specific ways of being with ourselves and others. These orientations have deeply influenced notions of wellbeing, our relationality to one another, and expectations of ourselves and society.

Knowing

How we exist in the world is interwoven with how we know the world. Modern Western subjectivity emerged from the forces of nationalism, extractive capitalism, and settler colonialism which constructed reality as linear and binary. The belief in the limitless possibility of progress was largely borne out by the imperial experience of the Scientific Revolution, which saw ever-expanding markets and categories of knowledge. However, Western knowledge revealed its moral and ethical limitations when dealing with the consequences of unrestricted colonization, eventually resulting in a fragmented sense of Western subjectivity uneasily existing in a perilous world. Here we look at what these kinds of subjectivity imply for ways of knowing the world, especially at the intersection of social wellbeing and health.

Educational and social and health care institutions in the Global North are based on the assumption that only Western scientific discourses can speak with power and authority about the nature of reality. However, our definitions of science are often embedded in social contexts that reproduce exclusions and invisibilities. Indigenous knowledges (as well as the knowledge of peoples from other disqualified groups such as ethnic minorities, disabled people, women, and sexual and gender minorities) have often been coalesced into categories such as 'folk belief systems,' 'street knowledge,' or 'old wives' tales' that have held lesser value in the eyes of the patriarchs of Western science (Kovach, 2009). Dismissive generalizations have ignored and rendered invisible many of the great scientific achievements of humankind such as the astronomical calculations of the Aztecs, the botanical knowledge of female midwives, and the medical knowledge of the ancient Egyptians. Western ways of knowing are deeply influenced by the twin structures and ideologies of extractive capitalism and settler colonialism.

People around the globe throughout time have observed the natural universe to understand how the world works – and all of their research, not just that of Western Europeans, was empirical. The Aztecs had complex understandings of astronomy, ancient Islamic scholars developed the principles of algebra and geometry, the Chinese developed the compass, gunpowder, and paper, while smallpox vaccinations were understood by West Africans long before they were introduced to the West (Waldstreicher, 2004). Before the rise of the persecuting society, many ancient Europeans also studied natural phenomena constructing Neolithic monuments such as Newgrange in Ireland and Stonehenge in England, which precisely captures the light of the winter solstice alignment. Scientific methods widely used in Indigenous societies around the globe predated the Scientific Revolution in the West.

Following Moore's argument (2009) that the persecuting society in Europe arose due to the centralization of power rather than the will of the masses, independent grassroots scientific investigation was often seen by rulers as heresy promoted by members of stigmatized groups and profoundly threatening to the social order. The emergence of the seventeenth-century Scientific Revolution signaled a rupture with the Church in matters of understanding and explaining the world and made Europeans more curious about how the world worked (Howe, 1994, 514).

The findings of Copernicus, Brahe, Newton, Kepler, and Galileo revolutionized Europeans' conception of themselves in the universe, ushering in new ways of constructing knowledge through empirical observation. Modern Western science emerged with a methodology that sought to comprehend the workings of the universe through a finite set of natural laws (Lipe, 2013, 118). Based on an individualistic sense of subjectivity, Western science viewed the world through the lens of sets of theorems that required empirical evidence to prove whether they were true. The scientific method held that nothing was true unless it could be proved through systematic data collection with replicable findings. Analysis was accomplished through dividing the problem into parts and understanding how each part worked separately and together. The use of these methods was key to understanding natural selection and genetics, the discovery of penicillin, the building of skyscrapers and bridges, and many other areas that have extended our lives and enriched their quality. At the same time, these methods often obscured holistic and spiritual understandings of human beings and their experience in the environment.

When Europeans moved into the modern era, they began to examine how to conceptualize society and construct notions of civilization in a changing time. The period between the fourteenth and eighteenth centuries has often been characterized in history books as the Age of Discovery. This period was framed as a religious mission by a series of papal bulls, also collectively referred to as the Doctrine of Discovery, issued between 1455 and 1493, which gave full and free permission with a Christian blessing for Europeans to colonize, commit genocide, and enslave non-Christian people and take their land (Wilkins and Lomawaima, 2001). During this time, Europeans utilized innovative seafaring and navigational technology as well as improved weaponry to travel far from their continent to invade other places around the world in search of spices, gold, and land to fuel rapidly industrializing European cities. For example, the Spanish pillaged more than 45,000 tons of pure silver from Potosi, Bolivia, between 1556 and 1783 (Kamen, 2004). Emerging industrial capitalism required a vast labor force. Hence, the brutal transatlantic slave trade was initiated to corral captive workers from Africa, Indigenous Peoples were pushed off land and often enslaved, and displaced rural communities in Europe began to flood into cities to produce goods manufactured from raw materials plundered from colonies. The scientific method thus shaped and was shaped by the sense of religious mission that drove settler colonialism and extractive capitalism. Power has always driven the resources available to scientific endeavors, continually reproducing an uneasy relationship between justice, truth, domination, and oppression.

The science of society has its roots in the methodologies of the Scientific Revolution, the racism of settler colonial ways of understanding the self and society, and the social disruption of the Industrial Revolution. There was a fierce debate at the end of the eighteenth century over whether Western civilization emanated from Greece or "the Orient." Philosophers who constructed much of the Western canon of knowledge, such as Immanuel Kant and Wilhelm Gottfried Tennemann, systematically erased Asian, Indigenous, and African scientific contributions, thus decisively reinforcing Eurocentrism as a core principle of Western constructions of knowledge (Park, 2013). Positivism, the scientific method of verifying assertions by empirical proof, was applied to ways of understanding society yet often without a social context. Auguste de Comte, often considered the founder of Western sociology, held that the only authentic knowledge is scientific (Heilbron, 1990). By this, he meant that facts must be substantiated by observable and documentable proof. Underlying this view is the assumption that knowledge is a direct perception of reality and therefore can be universalized. This orientation to knowledge also holds that reality can be objectively known by the subject. The holder of this 'objective knowledge' can thus assert authority and power over any other non-verifiable versions.

The Western divide between holistic mind–body and materialist–physical views of knowledge runs deep historically (Andersen, 2001). Reductionist views of science hold that complex phenomena can be distilled into their constituent elements, which are often based on material or empirical proof. Much of contemporary Western medical science, for example, is constructed on the foundation of reductionism addressing rather narrow conceptions of disease processes rather than the more complex dynamics of multifaceted personal and community issues that impact health status (Chummun, 2006).

Emerging sociological knowledge fixed its gaze on the future, seeking to develop new ways of knowing, understanding, and predicting society. As the Industrial Revolution progressed, many sociologists observed the paradox that as material wealth grew in the West and society became increasingly integrated through modern instruments such as schools, work, and the military, people nonetheless suffered from greater alienation and anomie in society. The work of Friedrich Engels documented the suffering of English workers during the Industrial Revolution (Engels, 1984). Noting that the political and social structures of society are grounded in its economy, Engels and Marx pointed out that as people were increasingly commodified through industrialized work and thus unable to make choices about their own lives and destinies, they inevitably became alienated from themselves, others, and their societies. Change, in the eyes of Engels and Marx, could only come when workers would seize the means of production and transform society. Emile Durkheim, a French Jew, focused his early sociological studies on social solidarity (Durkheim, 1964). He held that as modern societies became rapidly integrated and changed, people inevitably became more interdependent, though paradoxically, many people also experience a growing sense of disconnection or anomie. The more labor is specialized, Durkheim argued, the less connection people feel toward one another. Hence, an overriding social ideology or common social bond must be created to ensure the stability of social solidarity.

In the early twentieth century, modern sociological theory focused on social structures often through the lens of conflict or functionalism. Modernism sought to develop grand narratives to explain the interconnection of social structures and human agency. The Frankfurt School, for example, used critical theory as a tool to transform social science into a liberatory force (Wiggershaus, 1994). By integrating all forms of social sciences (e.g., geography, political science, sociology, and psychology), critical theorists focused on the historical specificity of societies in the attempt to understand how societies were uniquely configured materially and culturally. Critical theorists Theodor Adorno and Max Horkheimer argued that all theory must explain what's wrong with the current reality, identify what needs to change, and offer practical solutions for social transformation (Adorno and Horkheimer, 2016). However, thinkers such as Herbert Spencer and Talcott Parsons had a more pessimistic view of the possibilities of social liberation (e.g., Parsons and Mayhew, 1982; Spencer, 1879). They viewed social structures as entities composed of complex interconnected parts that continually seek equilibrium, ultimately constraining people's choices and actions.

In the postmodern era of the 1970s, social theorists increasingly challenged the foundations of modernist Western social science. They were critical of the role of science in collaborating with power. French philosopher Michel Foucault, for example, saw modern rationality as a coercive force that maintained discipline in society (Foucault and Rabinow, 2010). Through historical examinations of the birth of prisons, asylums, and clinics, Foucault explored how knowledge and practice have become part of a cultural matrix of power relations. Modern social science sought to understand how humanity was integrated into the emerging modern industrial society. Following the methods of natural science, social science attempted to generalize laws about reality and categorize the different qualities of reality. In the postmodern era, the intersection of power and knowledge was no longer seen as neutral but rather as reproducing oppressive relations. Social science thus became an increasingly contested terrain between those who sought to preserve its 'objective' empirical mission and those who viewed it as a means to challenge power structures and liberate society.

Some social science theorists think that we have entered a 'post-truth' era as a consequence of the symmetry of truths in postmodernism (Sismondo, 2017). Postmodernism opened up and recognized the multiple, complex perspectives on expertise that were often subordinated and marginalized, but the uncertainty of science has also been mobilized to argue against definitive facts on climate crisis, for example. Fujimura and Holmes (2019, 1251–1252) ask: "After spending several decades resisting uncritical acceptance of scientific authority and studying the production of scientific authority, should we now *resist* the *resistance* to scientific authority?" While reducing the hierarchies of knowledge has democratized ways of knowing by challenging traditional institutions, it has also ushered in increasing authoritarianism, trolling, and appeals to emotionalism instead of examining evidence. The emergence of post-truth culture has also fueled hectoring and stigmatizing judgements about the reasons for social exclusion, poverty, and other social issues, which has broad implications for how social work constructs and communicates knowledge and advocates for the most vulnerable.

Acting

Each historical era has a distinct social order that reflects how institutions, cultures, and values shape and are shaped by people's ways of interacting and behaving. The ancient Irish epic *Táin Bó Cúailnge* (*The Cattle Raid of the Cooley*), for example, paints a picture of an honor-based society rooted in reciprocity (O'Donnell, 2015). The *siida* system of the Sámi people in Northern Europe is a group-based system of democratic governance that structures cooperation in managing land rights and the environment to work with foraging reindeer (Hausner, Fauchald, Jernsletten, and Bawa, 2012). These types of societies reinforced the centrality of the collective in governing and stewarding shared resources in relationality with fellow creatures as well as supporting one another. However, a modern social space of alienation and distress emerged from the tectonic shifts of settler colonialism, the disruption of the Industrial Revolution, and the dispossession of many from their traditional ways of life, creating a rupture between human beings and their environment.

The loss of the commons at the dawn of the Industrial Revolution represented a fundamental shift away from a shared governance of resource management and communal space. As settler colonialism grew throughout the world, the commons, which were long seen in the words of early American revolutionary Tom Paine as "natural property, or that which comes to us from the Creator of the universe – such as the earth, air, water," were increasingly monopolized and consumed by individuals for private gain (Lamb, 2017, 133). The environment became a resource to plunder rather than one to nurture. The communal space of society was thus fragmented into parcels of private property.

The modern era constructed a social space that existed "between the private and the public, a field defined by both welfare and legal judgements, where interpersonal concerns are played out before a political audience" (Howe, 1994, 517). In other words, the state became involved in creating policies subject to prevailing political winds and forms of oppressions that defined what a family is, how the rights of children are understood, and how gender is performed. The reach of the state could be enormous, as Susan Schweik (2009) documents in her book *The Ugly Laws: Disability in Public*, showing how local laws in the United States criminalized and pathologized those considered 'diseased,' 'deformed,' or 'unsightly.' 'Ugly laws' were a series of ordinances starting in the late nineteenth century that outlawed 'unsightly begging.' Emerging in rapidly urbanizing cities subject to an influx of often needy new residents and injured Civil War soldiers, ugly laws sought to reinforce the normalizing standards of existing communities. The laws were shaped by prevailing notions of eugenics, race, class and gender, charity, institutionalization, and the appropriate designs of beautiful cities. According to Schweik (2009, 6), the last known prosecution of an individual under ugly laws occurred in Omaha, Nebraska, in 1974 when a homeless man was detained by police because he had "marks and scars" on his body. The case was later thrown out by the court.

The social professions emerged in complex and heterogeneous forms throughout the Western world at the turn of the twentieth century. Guided by scientific knowledge and legitimized by the state, the social professions generally embarked on one of two distinct paths that persist today (Rothman and Mizrahi, 2014). One route was more ideological and community oriented. It sought to challenge some of the most egregious aspects of industrial capitalism. Many of these practitioners focused on demanding social change on a spectrum ranging from radical to reformist viewpoints. Others began creating enormously complex systems of diagnosis to map the wide range of behaviors and identities deemed abnormal or troublesome. Some of the social professions were tasked by the state with 'normalizing' populations to provide a docile workforce for the needs of settler colonial extractive capitalism. Invested with statutory powers, the social professions often became agents of state control by enforcing heteronormative notions of the family; removing children from homes considered unsuitable according to racist, classist, ableist, and ethnocentric definitions of well-being; and labeling people who resisted the dominant social order as deviant (McDonald, 2014).

As one of the first proponents of professionalizing direct social work practice, Mary Richmond is often seen as a forerunner of the contemporary clinical orientation. Richmond argued that professionalized social work could deflect the mass appeal of socialism in the contentious atmosphere of industrial labor unrest and defend societal institutions (Reisch, 2016). Richmond's conception of social work as individualized helping that guided people toward a desired outcome as defined by the professional contradicts Indigenous ways of understanding solidarity and support for distressed individuals as a shared and equal relationship. Richmond's focus on training for clinical practice would lay the basis for the rise of professional associations that delineated the necessary qualifications and competencies to practice social work, creating a colonial relationship between experts and community. Professional associations are in many ways exemplars of settler colonial structures and processes. They maintain strict gatekeeping of qualifications and definitions of competence, are often expensive to join, and create dividing lines between those designated as 'professional helpers' and those not seen as qualified to help. Professional associations guard access to work opportunities, policymaking capacity, and resources.

The disempowerment of collective and community healing through the rise of social professionalism often created systems that alienated people from their identities and cultures, isolated individuals from community support, and disrupted traditional communal forms of connection, caring and healing. The early social work movement that began in the mid-nineteenth century America had little to do with Indigenous Peoples. Following the so-called Plains Indian Wars of the mid-1800s, many Indigenous Peoples became the wards of the federal government, whose main goal was to 'civilize' them so that they could assimilate into mainstream settler society. In 1897, Colonel Richard Henry Pratt, a veteran of the Civil War, established the first off-reservation Indian boarding school at Carlisle, Pennsylvania. Indian boarding schools were created to educate and assimilate Native children according to white settler standards. Pratt's goal was to "kill the Indian and save the man" (Churchill, 2004). Conditions on many Indian reservations at this time were dreadful. Indian leaders were disarmed, jailed, and isolated, and many tribes faced starvation, poverty, racism, sickness, disease, and high mortality. Tribes were no longer able to resist the control and domination of the United States. While they were at their weakest, Christian missionaries and the federal government began taking Indian children, against the will of the families, and sent them to off-reservation boarding schools hundreds of miles away. (This is similar to the Trump administration's current policy of family separation at the US southern border, which has resulted in thousands of children, some as young as four months old, removed from their parents. Crowded into facilities, several children have died from ailments, and there have been many accusations of physical, emotional, and sexual abuse). In the boarding schools, Native American children experienced many types of abuse, starvation, disease, and death. In the end, some of the children never made it home, while others who did were changed forever. Generally speaking, Pratt and the federal government, with the complicity of the fields of social work and education, were largely successful in killing the culture, language, dignity, and identity of Native Americans. Sámi children in Finland, Norway, and Sweden; First Nations children in Canada; and "half-cast" aboriginal children in Australia were also removed from their communities and sent to Christian and government boarding schools, facing many of the same draconian measures.

Social work has failed Indigenous communities because it is grounded in the epistemological foundation of settler colonial modernist science, which the profession uses to construct ways of defining and solving social problems (Payne and Askeland, 2008, 1). The discipline of social work has developed distinct ways of looking at the connection between society and the individual, including the person-in-environment paradigm, biopsychosocial perspectives, empowerment and advocacy, and how government relates to its citizenry. Yet social work knowledge largely retains a "professional imperialism," in the words of James Midgely (2008), that reinforces the privileging of a modernist Western view of social organization and social transformation in social work theory. Despite centering social justice as the basis of the social work profession, there have been tensions surrounding what it means to be a social work professional and how universal social work values are constructed and applied. Contemporary social work codes of ethics and practice competencies are based on Western notions of universality, human rights, sometimes narrow definitions of what constitutes social work knowledge, thus implicitly legitimating settler colonialism. Disproportionality in child protection is one example of how ethnic minority and Indigenous children are often seen as being in problematic situations requiring state intervention, raising questions of how social workers ethically manage risk, parental behaviors, and diverse cultures in systems based on settler colonialism.

Education is, as Ashcroft, Griffiths, and Tiffin (1995, 425) have noted, a formidable weapon in the arsenal of empire. In 1973, the American Council on Social Work Education stated for the first time that issues related to racial and ethnic minorities should be reflected in the social work curriculum, which was expanded in the 1980s to include issues related to ageism, sexism, and social and cultural diversity (Alvarez-Hernandez and Choi, 2017). Defined as "a set of congruent behaviors, attitudes, and policies that come together in a system, agency, or among professionals and enable the system, agency, or those professionals to work effectively in cross-cultural situations" (Cross, Bazron, and Dennis, 1989, iv), cultural competence emerged in the social work curriculum during the 1980s to instill professional awareness, skills, and behaviors for working with diverse populations. However, cultural competence has been criticized for not having clear and measurable ways of assessing mastery that can be distinguished from self-identity and years of professional experience (Larson and Bradshaw, 2017). Cultural competence reflects the strong aspiration of the social work profession to support diverse populations, but most research has focused on interventions with specific populations rather than demonstrating a global change in social work education (Nadan, 2017). Notions of cultural competence, for example, rarely analyze how social work is the product of the intersection of modernity and colonialism or how the practice of social work itself should change (McDonald, 2014). Hence, the social work frameworks passed down to emerging professionals through higher education remain informed by the colonial gaze of Western subjectivity and education, often diminishing the self-knowledge, cultural strengths, and collective healing of communities while enforcing colonized notions of individual recovery and wellness.

Evidence-based practice has become a cornerstone of social work in recent decades and a core value driving social policymaking (Haskins and Baron, 2015). It is seen as the latest best practice to utilize the concept of value-free empirical knowledge from the perspective of the expert to demonstrate the effectiveness of social and healthcare programs. By setting up various agencies to compete with one another for funding by comparing outcomes, evidence-based practice can enforce a boilerplate template for action driven by a neoliberal agenda of treatment-focused interventions with minimal dialogue or focus on the needs and perspectives of diverse communities (McDonald, 2014, 162).

A profession generally practiced as a statutory activity, social work has often been complicit with oppressive and hierarchical policies and practices. Some are starting to question the clinical-community binary and demand social work approaches that reflect a capacity to confront and redress the legacy of colonialism. In *Decolonizing Social Work*, the first comprehensive volume on the topic, Gray, Coates, Yellow Bird, and Hetherington (2016, xxi–xxii) argue,

> [Social work] must confront the continuing effects of colonialism and the ways in which the profession has been, and continues to participate in colonizing projects. . . . The decolonization of social work requires that the profession acknowledges its complicity in these unjust practices, ceases its participation in processes that disadvantage Indigenous Peoples, condemns the past and continuing effects of colonialism, and collaborates with Indigenous Peoples to engage in decolonizing actions against multinational companies, professional organizations, public agencies, and private not-for-profit projects.

In calling for a deeper reflection and analysis on how social work education continues to reproduce colonialism, Gray, Coates, Yellow Bird, and Hetherington (2016) demand concrete action to challenge the many ways that social work knowledge and practice is structured. Though anti-oppressive social work practices have evolved along with a number of other approaches, such as structural social work, critical social work, radical social work, feminist social work, and antiracist social work, to "minimize power hierarchies" and "to build the power of those who hold a marginalized identity and/or reducing the unfair power of those of privileged status" (Dominelli and Campling, 2014, 9), a decolonized social work practice would argue that this is not sufficient. None of these approaches specifically engages with decolonizing social work since they are settler approaches – radical approaches but settler approaches nonetheless.

Decolonizing social work seeks to transform a profession based on Western modernist scientific traditions so that it can divest itself of the oppressive ways of thinking and subsequent practices that have prevented social work from fulfilling its mission of enhancing well-being for all. It starts from the recognition that Indigenous Peoples have been the subjects (and victims) of the colonizing activities of settler structures and processes and that the goals of settler colonialism have included the elimination, manipulation, control, and replacement of the Native. Decolonization concerns the "repatriation of Indigenous land and life; it is not a metaphor for other things we want to do to improve our societies and schools" (Tuck and Yang, 2012, 1). Decolonizing social work, therefore, is not about advancing or employing settler social work approaches. Second, mainstream social work must acknowledge the limitations of Western knowing and imperialist models of practice that have damaged Indigenous Peoples and other communities (Gray, Coates, Yellow Bird, and Hetherington, 2016, 6). Finally, it must actively engage with and repair the damage done by the many years of complicity with settler colonial domination. Across the world, examples of decolonizing social work practice have begun to emerge: forest therapy in Sámi territory, trauma informed approaches to healing intergenerational trauma in Aboriginal

Australia, Indigenous healers working with mental health in rural India. Some of the commonalities of these approaches include a sensitivity and humility toward Indigenous and local ways of being and knowing (Gray, Coates, and Yellow Bird, 2008).

The underlying dilemma in providing care for Sunya and Yer lay precisely in the narrow focus of social and health interventions. Services were concentrated solely on ensuring that the women took the medicine, without considering the historical trauma and the complex relational context of the women's lives. Constructing an intervention in isolation from the equally important aspects of patients' lifeworlds is typical of settler colonial approaches. As we have seen in this chapter, the arc of Western subjectivity, knowledge, and action has bent toward compartmentalization, fragmentation, and partiality. How can we heal by only taking into account one part of our lives?

References

Adorno, T. W., and Horkheimer, M. 2016. *Dialectic of Enlightenment*. London: Verso.

Althusser, L. 2016. *Lenin and Philosophy and Other Essays*. Delhi: Aakar Books.

Alvarez-Hernandez, L. R., and Choi, Y. J. 2017. Reconceptualizing Culture in Social Work Practice and Education: A Dialectic and Uniqueness Awareness Approach. *Journal of Social Work Education*, 53(3): 84–398.

Andersen, H. 2001. The History of Reductionism versus Holistic Approaches to Scientific Research. *Endeavour*, 25(4): 153.

Anderson, B. 2006. *Imagined Communities: Reflections on the Origin and Spread of Nationalism*. New York: Verso.

Ashcroft, B., Griffiths, G., and Tiffin, H. 1995. *The Post-Colonial Studies Reader*. London: Routledge.

Bell, J. M. 2014. *The Black Power Movement and American Social Work*. New York: Columbia University Press.

Bender, D. E. 2008. Perils of Degeneration: Reform, the Savage Immigrant, and the Survival of the Unfit. *Journal of Social History*, 42(1), 5–29, 253.

Berenson, E., Duclert, V., and Prochasson, C. 2011. *The French Republic: History, Values, Debates*. Ithaca, NY: Cornell University Press.

Bullard, K. S. 2015. *Civilizing the Child: Discourses of Race, Nation, and Child Welfare in America*. Lanham: MD: Lexington Books.

Chummun, H. 2006. Reductionism and Holism in Coronary Heart Disease and Cardiac Nursing. *British Journal of Nursing*, 15(18): 1017–1020.

Churchill, W. 2004. *Kill the Indian, Save the Man: The Genocidal Impact of American Indian Residential Schools*. San Francisco: City Lights.

Cooper, F., and Stoler, A. 1997. *Tensions of Empire: Colonial Cultures in a Bourgeois World*. Berkeley: University of California Press.

Cross, T., Bazron, B., and Dennis, K. 1989. *The Cultural Competence Continuum: Toward a Culturally Competent System of Care: A Monograph on Effective Services for Minority Children Who Are Severely Emotionally Disturbed*. Washington, DC: Georgetown University Child Development Center.

Dominelli, L., and Campling, J. 2014. *Anti-Oppressive Social Work Theory and Practice*. Basingstoke: Palgrave Macmillan.

Durkheim, É. 1964. *The Division of Labor in Society*. New York: Free Press of Glencoe.

Engels, F. 1984. *The Condition of the Working Class in England*. London: Lawrence & Wishart.

Fanon, F. 1963. *The Wretched of the Earth*. New York: Grove Press.

Foucault, M., and Rabinow, P. 2010. *The Foucault Reader*. New York: Vintage.

Franklin, D. L. 1986. Mary Richmond and Jane Addams: From Moral Certainty to Rational Inquiry in Social Work Practice. *Social Service Review*, 60(4): 504–525.

Fraser, N. 2013. *Fortunes of Feminism: From State-managed Capitalism to Neoliberal Crisis*. London: Verso.

Froese, P., and Bader, C. 2008. Unraveling Religious Worldviews: The Relationship between Images of God and Political Ideology in a Cross-Cultural Analysis. *The Sociological Quarterly*, 49(4): 689–718.

Fujimura, J. H., and Holmes, C. J. 2019. Staying the Course: On the Value of Social Studies of Science in Resistance to the "Post-Truth" Movement. *Sociological Forum*, 34(S1): 1251–1263.

Gray, M., Coates, J., and Yellow Bird, M. (eds.). 2008. *Indigenous Social Work Around the World: Towards Culturally Relevant Education and Practice*. Aldershot: Ashgate.

Gray, M., Coates, J., Yellow Bird, M., and Hetherington, T. (eds.). 2016. *Decolonizing Social Work*. London: Routledge.

Harari, Y. 2015. *Sapiens: A Brief History of Humankind*. New York: Harper.

Haskins, R., and Baron, J. 2015. The Obama Administration's Evidence-Based Policy Initiatives: An Overview. *Brookings Institution*. Accessed 23 May 2018 at www.brookings.edu/~/media/research/files/articles/2011/4/obama-social-policy-haskins/04_obama_social_policy_haskins.pdf.

Hausner, V., Fauchald, P., Jernsletten, J., and Bawa, K. 2012. Community-Based Management: Under What Conditions Do Sámi Pastoralists Manage Pastures Sustainably? *Community-Based Management of Pastoral Ecosystems*, 7(12): E51187.

Heilbron, J. 1990. Auguste Comte and Modern Epistemology. *Sociological Theory*, 8(2): 153–162.

Hounmenou, C. 2012. Black Settlement Houses and Oppositional Consciousness. *Journal of Black Studies*, 43(6): 646–666.

Howe, D. 1994. Modernity, Postmodernity and Social Work. *British Journal of Social Work*, 24(5): 513–532.

Jarvis, C. 2006. Function versus Cause: Moving Beyond Debate. *Praxis*, 6(3): 44–49.

Kamen, H. 2004. *Empire: How Spain Became a World Power, 1492–1763*. New York: Perennial.

Kovach, M. 2009. *Indigenous Methodologies*. Toronto: University of Toronto.

Lamb, R. 2017. *Thomas Paine and the Idea of Human Rights*. Cambridge: Cambridge University Press.

Larson, K. E., and Bradshaw, C. P. 2017. Cultural Competence and Social Desirability among Practitioners: A Systematic Review of the Literature. *Children and Youth Services Review*, 76: 100.

Lipe, D. 2013. *Diversifying Science: Recognizing Indigenous Knowledge Systems as Scientific Worldviews*. PhD dissertation. University of Hawai'i – Manoa.

López-Ruiz, C. 2010. *When the Gods Were Born: Greek Cosmogonies and the Near East*. Cambridge, MA: Harvard University Press.

Margolin, L. 1997. *Under the Cover of Kindness: The Invention of Social Work*. Charlottesville: University Press of Virginia.

McDonald, C. 2014. *Challenging Social Work: The Institutional Context of Practice*. Basingstoke: Palgrave Macmillan.

McGrath, P. 2002. Early Medieval Irish Monastic Communities: A Premodern Model with Post-Modern Resonances. *Culture and Organization*, 8(3): 195–208.

Mencken, F. C., Bader, C., and Embry, E. 2009. In God We Trust: Images of God and Trust in the United States among the Highly Religious. *Sociological Perspectives*, 52(1): 23–38.

Midgely, J. 2008. Promoting Reciprocal International Social Work Exchanges: Professional Imperialism Revisited. In *Indigenous Social Work Around the World: Towards Culturally Relevant Education and Practice*, edited by M. Gray, J. Coates, and M. Yellow Bird, 31–45. Aldershot: Ashgate.

Moore, R. I. 2009. *The Formation of a Persecuting Society: Authority and Deviance in Western Europe, 950–1250*. Malden, MA: Blackwell.

Nadan, Y. 2017. Rethinking "Cultural Competence" in International Social Work. *International Social Work*, 60(1): 74–83.

O'Donnell, L. 2015. *On the Edge of the Cauldron: Identifying a Shamanic Paradigm in Celtic Culture*. PhD dissertation. Saybrook University.

Park, P. K. 2013. *Africa, Asia, and the History of Philosophy: Racism in the Formation of the Philosophical Canon, 1780–1830*. SUNY Series, Philosophy and Race. Albany: State University of New York Press.

Parsons, T., and Mayhew, L. 1982. *Talcott Parsons on Institutions and Social Evolution: Selected Writings*. Heritage of Sociology. Chicago: University of Chicago Press.

Payne, M., and Askeland, G. A. 2008. *Globalization and International Social Work: Postmodern Change and Challenge*. London: Ashgate.

Percovich, L. 2004. Europe's First Roots: Female Cosmogonies Before the Arrival of the Indo European Peoples. *Feminist Theology*, 13(1): 26–39.

Reisch, M. 2016. Why Macro Practice Matters. *Journal of Social Work Education*, 52(3): 258–268.

Rodriguez Garcia, E. 2011. The Challenge of Cultural Diversity in Europe: (Re)designing Cultural Heritages Through Intercultural Dialogue. *Human Architecture: Journal of the Sociology of Self-Knowledge*, 9(4): 49–60.

Rothman, J., and Mizrahi, T. 2014. Balancing Micro and Macro Practice: A Challenge for Social Work. *Social Work*, 59(1): 91–93.

Schech, S., and Haggis, J. 2002. *Development: A Cultural Studies Reader*. Malden, MA: Blackwell.

Schwartz, A. 1999. Americanization and Cultural Preservation in Seattle's Settlement House: A Jewish adaptation of the Anglo-American Model of Settlement Work. *Journal of Sociology & Social Welfare*, 26(3): 25–47.

Schweik, S. M. 2009. *The Ugly Laws: Disability in Public*. New York: New York University.

Sismondo, S. 2017. Post-truth? *Social Studies of Science*, 47(1): 3–6.

Spencer, H. 1879. *Social Structures*. New York: Appleton.

Spivak, G. C. 2010. Can the Subaltern Speak?: Revised Edition, from the "History" Chapter of Critique of Postcolonial Reason. In *Can the Subaltern Speak?: Reflections on the History of an Idea*, edited by Rosalind, 21–78. New York: Columbia University Press.

Trattner, W. I. 1998. *From Poor Law to Welfare State: A History of Social Welfare in America*. 6th ed. New York: Free Press.

Tuck, E., and Yang, K. W. 2012. Decolonization Is Not a Metaphor. *Decolonization: Indigeneity, Education & Society*, 1(1): 1–40.

Türken, S., Nafstad, H. E., Blakar, R. M., and Roen, K. 2016. Making Sense of Neoliberal Subjectivity: A Discourse Analysis of Media Language on Self-Development. *Globalizations*, 2015: 32-46.

Vang, T. 1979. Racial and Cultural Variations among American Families: A Decennial Review of Literature on Minority Families. *Journal of Marriage and the Family*, 42: 887–904.

Waldstreicher, D. 2004. *Runaway America: Benjamin Franklin, Slavery, and the American Revolution*. New York: Hill and Wang.

Wiggershaus, R. 1994. *The Frankfurt School: Its History, Theories, and Political Significance*. Cambridge, MA: MIT Press.

Wilkins, D. E., and Lomawaima, K. T. 2001. *Uneven Ground: American Indian Sovereignty and Federal Law*. Norman, OK: University of Oklahoma Press.

2 Postcolonial trauma and memory work

MICHAEL SHARES A STORY

I, Michael, want to share an important teaching that I learned from one of our revered spiritual tribal elders. People often think trauma only happens to humans and perhaps to animals. But many Indigenous Peoples believe that trauma can become embedded in all forms of life. Trauma has been clinically defined as a deeply distressing or disturbing experience that exists along a complex spectrum affecting childhood development with lifelong emotional and physical consequences (Briere and Spinazzola, 2005). Trauma is the result of a high level of stress that stretches beyond the mind's capacity to process new information, overwhelming the individual's ability to act and feel (Herman, 2015). Today, trauma studies, theories, and approaches such as trauma-informed care and adverse childhood experiences research, are widely in use within the human services professions to better understand the mechanisms of trauma and how they might be mediated and healed.

I have found that within Indigenous communities, trauma has a much larger context which goes far beyond the individual human and group. Indigenous Peoples' traditional beliefs throughout the world have generally agreed that all things, rocks, earth, lands, plants, trees, waters, grasses, animals, and insects, are alive (sentient) and that humans have connections to them and hold obligations to each of these non-human beings and places – a conception that David Anderson (2000, 116) has referred to as "sentient ecology." While this concept is not new to Indigenous Peoples, anthropologist Timothy Ingold (2000, 25) frames these communicative relationships between humans and their environments beyond that of just knowledge, "based in feeling, consisting in the skills, sensitivities and orientations that have developed through long experience of conducting one's life in a particular environment." Studies indicate that plants possess a sentience that enables them to see, hear, smell, possess awareness, and respond (Chamovitz, 2017). Does the same hold for rocks, insects, waters, and lands? Indigenous Peoples certainly think so. Maybe, in time, non-Indigenous Peoples will discover this for themselves.

In the early 1990s, I was working on my PhD in the School of Social Welfare at the University of Wisconsin–Madison. During the summers, my sons and I would journey from Wisconsin back to our reservation in North Dakota to spend time with my mother and father (the grandparents) and our many relatives. It was also a time when my sons and I would reacquaint ourselves with our horses who were staying at my parents' farm. My father and mother both grew up around horses and used them to help with the chores on their farms and as a main source of recreation and transportation.

Horses hold a special place in my family, and many of my relatives have traditional tribal names that demonstrate our connection to horses. My second oldest son, Michael, was given the name 'Many Horses' by his grandfather (my father) My younger brother, Monte, carries the name 'Black Pinto Horse,' which he received during a sacred ceremony. My older brother, Dennis, a military veteran from the Vietnam War era, was given the name 'One of Many Horses.' My uncle, Leroy (Harold), my father's brother, was called 'Sky Horse' or 'Horse Above,' a very sacred name. My father and many of the older men in our community spoke often of our tribal belief that horses, like dogs, were very sensitive, spiritual creatures that had the power to sense things that humans could not.

One particular summer during our regular visit to my parents' farm, my second oldest son, Michael, and I received a very important traditional teaching about trauma that encompassed horses, humans, the lands, and many other non-human witnesses. We arrived at my parents' place late in the evening and made time to visit about riding our horses the next day. Then we called it a night and went to bed. The next morning, I was awakened by birds singing before the sun had risen and the smell of coffee and the early morning laughter and visiting of my family. I went into the kitchen and poured a cup of coffee and joined them to chat on the large, covered front porch of my parents' house and to enjoy "the sun rising on this" warm summer morning. My sons and nephews were already dressed, geared up, and ready to go ride.

As we drove down to the lands where the horses were located, we discussed what our father had told us the day before about how we must have a good sense of patience when we were reacquainting ourselves with our horses and any others that we might ride. Dad always told us to proceed in a manner that was friendly, relaxed, and calm so we didn't spook the horses or get them overly excited and make them difficult to handle. He always said to us: "Remember, that horses are a lot like people; they have emotions, fears, and can easily mistrust someone that abuses them or makes them afraid. You want to make sure that your horse knows what you expect from him." Along the way, we stopped for a while to watch a mother fox and her pups trotting in the plowed, dark fields, hunting mice, grasshoppers, and looking for bird nests on the ground.

When we arrived at our destination, we fathers and uncles began giving our sons and nephews our unsolicited advice about what to do and how they should handle their horses, which garnered us side glances, raised eyebrows, and polite silence. After a short time, they caught the horses and began gently rubbing them down, giving them treats to chew on, and saddling them up for the ride. The horse that my son had selected was a large, impressive muscular roan-colored quarter horse named 'Swede,' after Swede Johanson, the huge, formidable looking Marine in Clint Eastwood's 1986 movie *Heartbreak Ridge*. The horse had been ridden many times and was relaxed and cooperating and doing all that was asked of him. After some minor alterations of his gear, my son stepped up to Swede grabbed the saddle horn, put his left foot in the stirrup of the saddle, swung aboard, and squared himself in the saddle. Swede took a few steps and relaxed, waiting for the next cue. As he was settling himself, I hollered to Michael: "Double-check your stirrup length and make sure they fit your leg length. Be sure to talk to your horse and rub his neck before you get started. Let him get used to your and energy, and get off and lead him around the pen for just a minute." Everything looked fine with all our riders and horses, so we all proceeded in our trucks and on horseback to the river for a swim.

My brother and I drove ahead looking at the beautiful, green rolling hills, prairie dogs playing, and a few deer grazing upon tender summer plants just out-side a tree line. All of a sudden, Swede came barreling by without my son aboard. Shortly after he disappeared over the hill, one of the nephews quickly rode up to us and said: "Mike got thrown. He's okay but a little banged up. You guys go get him, and I'll catch his horse." We turned around and soon found Mike limping down the pasture road. We stopped and picked him up and asked if he was okay; I could see the hurt and worry in his eyes, but he replied: "I'm okay. What about my horse?" I pointed at my nephew Jeff, who was in the distance churning up dust as he was chasing down the horse. I said: "He should catch up with him pretty soon and bring him back."

To relieve Mike's worry, I said: "Swede was moving pretty quickly, so I'm sure he's fine." His uncle asked him what happened. "He got spooked when we were riding by that patch of trees" Mike replied. I asked him, "Was anyone else with you that might have seen anything that might have spooked him?" "No. It was just me," he said. "Their horses didn't want to go near those trees. They were all acting up when they came to that area."

After we were certain Mike was okay and Jeff had successfully caught and brought back Swede, we went back to where he was thrown to see if there were any hidden dangers the horses would have noticed and that we might have missed. We didn't find anything.

That evening after we got home and had some dinner that my mother had prepared, I grabbed a cup of coffee and sat down with my father to tell him had happened. He sat up in his chair, leaned forward, listened quietly, and then asked if the horse and Mike were both okay and what spooked Swede. I said we checked the area out, and we didn't see anything, but all our riders told us that all of their horses got anxious and fidgety when they were near that area. My father relaxed a bit, sat back, and said, "You better go see Sam and tell him what happened. Maybe there's something he could tell you." Sam was a well-known spiritual elder on our reserva-tion. He was also our Sun Dance chief and medicine man and had helped to heal a lot of the physical and spiritual sickness of many people on and off our rez. Sam was special. He was an individual unlike most of us. He was a solitary, prayerful man, who stayed very near his home and property, where he kept many ancient, sacred items that he used in his healing rituals. Over the years, I had spoken a number of times to Sam and came to deeply respect his knowledge, prophecies, intuitive abilities, and kindness towards people and animals. When he was a younger man, he had raised, cared for, and ridden many horses. He had an intimate knowledge about horses and people in both a practical and spiritual sense.

My father said, "He knows the ceremony that has to be done whenever someone is thrown from a horse. From what I understand, it helps to take care of whatever caused the horse to misbehave and takes away the experience from the rider, so that he doesn't carry it around with him."

Later on that night, I called Sam and explained what had happened and what my father had said. He told me to come to his place and to bring my son, Michael, with me. The next morning, we drove to Sam's house, which was a few hours away, on the other side of our reservation near the badlands. During the drive, Michael asked a number of questions about the ceremony his grandfather would perform and what the end result might be. I had no idea, and just to make sure that my attitude or ignorance would not influence my son's thinking, I told him I had never been a part of the ceremony and didn't know what to expect. The drive was pleasant and calming as we passed through the beautiful, ancient badlands where our people had once lived and, at times, isolated themselves on clay buttes to sit for long days of fasting and prayer. When we arrived, Sam was outside facing the north with his back to us, standing a distance from his house, deep in prayer. We waited for a moment in our car to allow him to finish, but he turned around and signaled us over, and with his permission, we stepped into the circle he was in. It was marked by long stems of sage that were interspersed with branches of cedar. As we entered his circle, he smudged us off and continued his prayers for a long, long time, talking to the clouds, winds, skies, lands, and the spirits that watch over us. We stood silently, listening carefully.

When he finished praying, we gently stepped out of the circle and walked back to his house and sat down at the kitchen table. He offered us a cup of tea made from a wild prairie flower called yellow coneflower, which he said was good for headaches and calmed a nervous stomach. We sipped the tea and talked for a while about the upcoming Sun Dance on our reservation and other ceremonies that would be held at different locations throughout the summer. When there was a lull in the conversation, Sam asked my son what had happened and why he thought the horse might have thrown him. Michael began sharing his story, carefully retracing the events starting with him catching the horse, saddling him up, and riding through the area where the horse became skittish and threw him off. Sam listened carefully, and when Mike had finished telling what happened, he asked a number of questions about the horse: what he looked like, how often he had been ridden, whether this behavior was typical for him, and any feelings that Mike may been having at the time of the ride. Mike answered all his queries, and finally, Sam, who had spent a lifetime understanding the dreamworld, asked him about any dreams that he had in the past few days.

Satisfied that he had enough information, Sam said, "Let's go back outside so we can wash away what happened to Mike so that he doesn't carry it with him the next time he goes riding. As we walked back out, I could feel that the cool morning had gone into hiding, and the early afternoon temperatures had risen considerably. All the birds that were singing and the insects that buzzing earlier that morning were now quiet.

We reentered the prayer circle that Sam had been standing in when we first arrived. He began with saying prayers to all the directions of the universe, and then started cleansing both Mike and I with a sweetgrass smudge and prayed as he waved the smoke over us. When he finished, he put his hands on my son's shoulders and faced him in the direction of where the incident had occurred. He began wiping down Mike with an eagle feather and a lock of horse hair and began singing a healing song in his tribal language as he lightly brushed his hair, eyes, face, ears, upper body, arms, back, chest, legs, and feet. When he finished, he stood behind him and put a hand on the back of his right shoulder and began a long prayer. A few tears rolled down his face as he prayed. I glanced away since his tears triggered my own tears as I suddenly realized that there were few elders left on our reservation who could do this ceremony, and one day Sam would pass, as would I, as would my son, as would the ceremony. When he was done, he stepped back and pulled a red handkerchief out of the back pocket of his dusty Levi's jeans and wiped his nose and face. Red is the color of protection.

Sam said, "Let's go back to the house and sit down. Mike, I want to tell you about the ceremony we just did." He repeated that the reason for doing the ceremony was to remove the negative energy and trauma from my son so that he would not be afraid to ride horses and that the horses would not be afraid of him. I thought we were finished, and I was going to give my thanks to Sam and Michael was about to give his grandfather some gifts he had brought for him. Sam turned away from us and began putting away the sacred articles that he had used and then said, "Now we have to go and wipe down the horse you were riding to take away the trauma that happened to him. Remember, he was also a part of what happened, and he needs to be cleaned off so that he doesn't carry this disturbance either."

We left Sam's and continued to visit and tell stories as we drove the long distance, back to our side of the reservation, to the place where the horse was corralled. At first, the horse moved away from us, appearing to be quite anxious and uneasy. I caught him and brought him over to Sam, who began talking softly to him in his traditional language and gently stroking the horse with his hand, which immediately calmed him down. He next brought out a small, hand-sized braid of sweetgrass and began to lightly rub down the horse as he prayed in his language. The horse smelled the sweetgrass and nibbled on it for a moment and then relaxed. Sam gently brushed his eyes, ears, nose, neck, and back and continued talking to the horse. Again, I thought we were finished.

Sam said, "Mike, take me to where this all happened." We drove down to the patch of trees and got off the truck. Sam walked into the center of the path that went through the trees. He looked around and then said, "Now we have to clean off this area and everything that witnessed what happened. Trauma is like a rock that is thrown into the water. It spreads itself out and can travel and get stuck in the land, trees, water, insects, leaves, rocks, and animals – all these things." Sam began talking to this place, slowly turning in a clockwise circle, acknowledging and speaking to everything he could see. He looked down and spoke to the earth, rocks, and grasses and any insects that were crawling nearby. Then he took out his smudge and began to gently wipe down some of the trees, leaves, and branches that had witnessed what had happened and spoke to them about letting go of what they had witnessed so that they were no longer afraid and affected. A few birds were sitting in branches near where we were. Sam spoke to them about what had happened and if they had witnessed it or their other bird relatives had witnessed it they should let go of what they had seen and experienced. He turned his attention to the ground and began wiping down the grasses, rocks, and place where he had been standing to help them release their memory of the trauma. With his eyes closed, he stood in silence for some minutes and then said, "Okay. All done."

We walked back to our truck and got in and drove away. In the rearview mirror, I could see the horse in the corral getting smaller and smaller. After a while, Sam said to me, "Mike, did your dad ever tell you about this ceremony?" "No," I replied. "When I told my dad what happened, he just said that you and a few others still know how to do the ceremony and that we should go and see you." We sat in silence for a while as we drove down the bumpy gravel road. Sam looked out his window and said, "Yeah. These ways are disappearing and will soon be gone. There's a lot of things that happen to the earth, the waters, and animals that we humans ignore. We focus only on ourselves. But the old people did not grow up that way. Our ancestors have always reminded us that we are connected to all things. Whatever causes harm to them causes harm to us. We feel their trauma, and they feel ours." We drove west towards the setting summer sun and before long we were driving silently in darkness.

Postcolonial trauma

The connection between settler colonialism and the present-day trauma of Indigenous Peoples and other oppressed populations is often denied. Acknowledging historical injustice requires action to confront the ongoing systems of oppression put in place by the original colonial violence (McGregor, 2012). In popular American culture, settler colonialism is often presented like an old artifact lurking in the closet of our national history like our grandfather's ancient military uniform: musty, a bit out of fashion, and vaguely heroic. The American history textbooks that we use to inculcate our young people with our national story rarely mentions the trauma that has been born of settler colonialism. Settler colonial systems of oppression and their corresponding practices have fundamentally shaped our ways of understanding ourselves, others, and our society. Even social work, which advocates strongly towards challenging oppression in all its forms as the defining mission of the field rarely addresses the legacy of the traumas associated with the Doctrine of Discovery and settler colonialism in its basic textbooks (Yellow Bird, 1999). Instead, many textbooks leap into the intersectional categories of race, ethnicity, gender, ability, and sexual identity with only the briefest of nods to the complex dimensions of settler colonialism. A major critique of trauma studies by postcolonial theorists is its Eurocentrism. The traumatic historical legacy of settler colonialism lives on in the material and ideological systems undergirding our current structure of privilege and oppression (Visser, 2011). As educator and bestselling author James Loewen has noted,

> The worshipful biographical vignettes of Columbus in our textbooks serve to indoctrinate students into a mindless endorsement of colonialism . . . the Columbus myth allows us to accept the contemporary division of the world into developed and underdeveloped spheres as natural and given, rather than a historical product issuing from a process that began with Columbus's first voyage.
>
> (2018, 70)

The power of the narrative of the Doctrine of Discovery as a benign activity is reflected in the fact that many Americans (including political leaders) do not believe the United States was involved in violent, traumatic settler colonial activities in the 'founding' of this nation. For instance, even the Harvard-educated, progressive supporter of Native American causes and first African American President Barack Obama argued in a 2009 interview with al-Arabiya Television that the United States could be an honest broker in the Israeli–Palestinian conflict. Obama said: "We sometimes make mistakes. We have not been perfect. But if you look at the track record, as you say, America was not born as a colonial power" (Gilgoff, 2009). Sadly, Obama's comments show complete disregard for the pain, losses, and traumas suffered by Indigenous Peoples in both past and present times. His statement reveals why there is a need for a postcolonial trauma theory that can fiercely interrogate the privileging traumas of white settlers while disenfranchising the suffering of Indigenous Peoples and other marginalized populations. In response to Obama's claims, Indigenous history professor and scholar Roxanne Dunbar-Ortiz (2009) pointed out that:

> The United States was founded as a European settler state, with maps and plans already prepared to colonize the continent coast to coast, expanding from the 13 colonies of the founding state. Indeed the US was the first state born as a colonial power, unique in the vast territories it brutally conquered, occupied, and administered, crushing over 300 indigenous nations, force-marching hundreds of thousands east of the Mississippi out of their homelands, crowding them into 'Indian Territory' (Oklahoma), along the way annexing half the Republic of Mexico.

Here Dunbar-Ortiz concisely lays out the breadth and depth of the violence of settler colonialism that is so casually denied by President Obama in his interview.

Some may ask: What does it matter if current President Donald Trump selects nineteenth-century president Andrew Jackson as the predecessor he most venerates? What does Andrew Jackson's legacy of Indigenous Peoples' genocide and African slave ownership have to do with the present United States? Why should statues of Confederate generals be removed from New Orleans? What does it matter if Indigenous Peoples have had long and deep connection from time immemorial to the Bears Ears National Monument in Utah when there are oil resources to exploit? Who cares if the money to found Ivy League colleges came from slave owners or that they are all built on stolen Indigenous Peoples' lands? All of this was a long time ago, so what does it have to do with now? How does the genocide of native peoples, enslavement of millions of Africans and Indigenous Peoples, and the confiscation of enormous portions of land continue to define the global sociopolitical and economic context in which we practice social work?

The structures that shape our lives are entwined with settler colonial ideologies and the extractive capitalist economy. Symbols of colonialism are strewn across the visual landscapes of North America and Europe. Recent global demonstrations protesting police violence and racism have pulled down or vandalized many statues of conquistadores, Confederate generals, and British imperialists in a resounding rejection of the continuing presence of symbols of the inhumanity of colonization in our everyday lives. Yet, colonialism continues to thrive through oppressive relationships in the form of racism, sexism, homophobia, ableism, and other ideologies which are infused in complex networks of power relations that maintain control through inequality, disunity, and injustice. Though the mission of social work explicitly seeks to change these power imbalances, its practices often individualize distress thus failing to address the settler colonial institutional cultures, environments, and patterns that allow discrimination and oppression to prosper. In this chapter, we discuss the historical emergence of the concept of trauma, then map out the historical socioeconomic development of the contemporary settler colonial landscape to provide a frame of reference for understanding the roots of postcolonial trauma and the role of memory in healing.

A historical progression of trauma

The settler colonial world was based on the rules and concepts of the seventeenth-century European Treaty of Westphalia, which established the notions of sovereignty, the equality of states, and territorial integrity. However, these principles were not applied to the multifarious nations of Indigenous Peoples encountered throughout the world by colonizers. The papal bull *Inter caetera* issued by Pope Alexander VI in the fifteenth century, for example, granted Spain and Portugal the moral right to kill, enslave, and take the land of non-Christians around the world. Papal bulls made conquest virtuous.

Prior to European colonization, there were substantial Indigenous civilizations around the world composed of empires with rulers of several states and kingdoms with single rulers and ruling families. There were also multitudes of smaller self-governing units, some affiliated with and controlled by the larger kingdoms and others existing in direct opposition to them. The Iroquois Confederacy, for example, comprised six great nations that utilized participatory democracy in shared governance. The Confederacy was centered around a matrilineal society that promoted gender equality and used the Great Law of Peace to address disputes and prevent warfare. Settler colonialism systematically destroyed these nations through divide-and-rule tactics, burning and looting, and genocide (Dunbar-Ortiz,

2014, 77). Colonial America eventually appropriated many of the symbols of the Iroquois Confederacy in the regalia of its emerging federal government. This cycle of ransacking resources, stealing land, and destroying communities and peoples, then hijacking and appropriating the symbols of the cultures in order to dilute their social and spiritual power, devastated Indigenous groups around the globe, and remains the modus operandi of many contemporary processes such as globalization and gentrification.

The confluence of the nation-state, modern systems of knowledge, and the extractive economy homogenized strategies and techniques of domination over diverse peoples across the globe. If the settler colonial world emerged from modern notions of sovereignty, democracy, citizenship, and human rights applied selectively to certain groups, then power elites in our contemporary neoliberal world use many of the same techniques of the extractive economy while hollowing out civic space and stripping social rights during a seemingly endless state of exception (Agamben, 2012). Settler colonial legacies continue to haunt and trouble global societies in complex ways. Their ideologies and material power have an impact on how knowledge and expertise are constructed, shaping societal understandings of what makes a good life, what role people should assume in society, and the value assigned to diverse human lives. So, to understand how social work as a contemporary intervention continues to replicate many of the roles of colonial subjectivity and domination – and then to further imagine how we might fundamentally transform the field as a vehicle for liberation – we must first unpack how the trauma of colonization continues to have an impact on individuals and communities.

Settler colonialism is not only an ideological structure but has a material power base. Between 1880 and 1914, most of the world outside Europe and North America was annexed and consolidated under the rule of a handful of European nations. The British Empire, for example, had dominion over a quarter of the world, containing at the time over 400 million subjects. The fortunes made through the displacement of Indigenous Peoples, the Atlantic slave trade, and the monopoly of the East India Company amounted to trillions of pounds and represented a massive transfer of wealth to the British. Divide-and-rule, ideologies of inferiority, and the devastation of local cultures were all tactics used by colonial powers to maintain domination of the colonized.

There is overwhelming evidence that settler colonialism took a tremendous toll on Indigenous Peoples (Dobyns and Swagerty, 1983; Dunbar-Ortiz, 2014; Stannard, 1992). Diseases such as malaria, smallpox, and typhus brought by European invaders killed nearly 90% of the Indigenous population of North America (McKenna and Pratt, 2015, 375). Tens of thousands of Native Americans died from enslavement, rivaling the number that perished from European infectious diseases (Reséndez, 2017). Fifteen to twenty million Africans were kidnapped into the Atlantic slave trade, and nearly one-fourth died during the terrible Middle Passage (Haines, McDonald, and Shlomowitz, 2001). Ten million people were murdered in the Congo during the vicious labor policies of King Leopold II of Belgium (Weisbord, 2003). Between 1845 and 1852, during the Great Famine in Ireland, one and a half million died and another million emigrated at the same time that the British colonial masters continued to export food to English markets (Mokyr and Grda, 2002). Anglo-Irish landlords evicted desperately impoverished Irish peasants and burned down their hovels, forcing millions to emigrate in coffin ships to the United States (Donnelly, 2001). African American slave children in the American South were shorter than 99% of non-enslaved American children and often suffered from night blindness, rickets, convulsions, and bowed legs due to undernourishment (Mintz, 2019). Tens of thousands of Indigenous Peoples have been removed from their lands and slaughtered as part of the process of settler colonialism. We can see this pattern from the nineteenth-century forced marches of the Chickasaw, Choctaw, and Cherokee to the twentieth-century stolen generations of Aboriginal Australians to the residents of Bikini Atoll displaced by US nuclear testing and the ongoing expulsion of Palestinians and Bedouin Arabs from their own lands. In all of these instances, the wrenching of people from their land has aimed at stealing resources and severing populations from their cherished sense of place and healing ceremonies that provide a sense of identity and connection. When considering the overwhelming numbers of casualties of settler colonialism, though, it is important to recall that each victim was not only emblematic of an oppressed social group but was also a beloved family and community member connected to a place. The sudden and traumatic rupture of these ties to one another and to the land reverberates down generations.

When it was created over 500 years ago by the Catholic Church, the body of law known as the Doctrine of Discovery gave dominion over all non-European land claimed by any European Christian nation that 'found' it (Miller, Ruru, Behrendt, and Lindberg, 2014). The 1452 Dum Diversas Bull issued by Pope Nicholas V stated that Portuguese King Alphonso V had the right "to capture, vanquish, and subdue the Saracens, pagans, and other enemies of Christ and put them into perpetual slavery and to take all their possession and their property" (Andrea and Neal, 2011). This doctrine was based on a Roman law which viewed all non-Christian land as terra nullius ("nobody's land"), interpreted to mean that all land unoccupied by European Christians was considered uninhabited and thus subject to sovereignty and title by any European Christian nation that 'discovered' it. Many of the principles of the Doctrine of Discovery are entrenched in Western property law. In 1823, for example, the US Supreme Court ruled in *Johnson v. McIntosh* that Indigenous People could not own or sell land (Watson, 2012). In 2005, the Doctrine of Discovery was cited as precedent in the case of the *City of Sherrill v. Oneida Indian Nation of New York* heard before the US Supreme Court (Berkey, 2005). In this case, the court ruled that even though the Oneida had purchased their original tribal lands because 200 years had elapsed between the initial dispossession and the purchase, the Oneida were not entitled to tribal sovereignty over the land.

The Doctrine of Discovery has had an impact on property laws beyond the Indigenous Peoples of North America. Lieutenant James Cook declared Australia to be terra nullius in 1770, which instigated its conquest by the British and the subsequent disenfranchisement of Australia's estimated 750,000 Indigenous Peoples (Igler, 2017). Though the concept of terra nullius was overturned, a 1992

Australian court decision reiterated that it accepted the British declaration of sovereignty over Australia in 1788 and the consequent body of Australian property law (Kramer, 2016). The Doctrine of Discovery thus resounds down through the generations across the globe, continuing to determine the legal relationship of people to place.

On the 4th of May 2016, a delegation of Indigenous Peoples from around the world converged as the March to Rome came to St. Peter's Square in the Vatican to demand the revocation of papal bulls authorizing the Doctrine of Discovery. These leaders called for Church recognition that the fifteenth-century papal bulls were responsible for the conquest of Indigenous territories and subsequent genocide and enslavement of Native peoples. Further, the March to Rome called for Vatican acknowledgement that contemporary human rights violations and ideologies of inequality have roots in the papal bulls. Pope Francis responded in a casual meeting with Dr. Kenneth Deer (Mohawk and Haudenosaunee representative) that he would pray for Indigenous Peoples (Long March to Rome, 2016).

The Doctrine of Discovery gave impetus to a colonial geographical project of mapping the world through exploration and conquest. The skill of cartography became a valuable asset for colonial powers to gain advantage over their European rivals, especially in conditions of war. As resources were identified, trade routes became established, and administrative institutions of control were put in place by settlers or colonial officials. These structures were enforced by the powerful militaries of empire that defended the global flow of resources from south to north. Settlers colonized and renamed New England, New Amsterdam, and Louisiana in the United States with Liverpool and New South Wales appearing in Australia while destroying ancient Indigenous landscapes. Toponymic inscription, the exercise of place naming, became an important tool of erasing Indigenous memory and exerting power over territory (Njoh, 2017). As European colonial dominance over the land, peoples, and resources of the world tightened, it became increasingly possible to rule other nations from home via complex global economic systems backed by the threat of military might and financial sanctions.

The era of the Doctrine of Discovery gradually transformed by the twentieth century from settler colonialism to imperialism (and eventually twenty-first century neoliberalism) through a complex global system that gradually outsourced the logistics of domination and resource extraction. Palestinian scholar Edward Said (1993, 9) defined imperialism as "the practice, the theory and the attitudes of a dominating metropolitan center ruling a distant territory." A crucial distinction between the two historical systems is that settler colonialism brings newcomers to dominate and brutally subjugate at the source of the extractive economy, where they remain and forge a new national identity while eradicating the natives. Imperialism, on the other hand, rules and manipulates from afar through economic and ideological means. At the height of the British Empire in India, for example, hundreds of provincial governments were under the direct rule of the British Viceroy and Governor General, who in turn carried out the will of the British government in London. Ruling the vast subcontinent of India from London was possible not only by military might but also through a complex web of administrative, ideological, and cultural structures that shaped local ways of governing and thinking. Colonization imposed artificial political borders, devastated local ways of living with the environment, and destroyed communities in the insatiable hunt for resources to wrest from distant lands and put in the service of the metropole. The shift from colonialism to imperialism reflected the increasing reluctance of empires to take responsibility for the administration of their territories in dealing with the needs of the local population. As dominant empires moved into the twentieth century, they sought to avoid enforcing direct rule over subject peoples while maintaining economic control over formerly colonized nations' natural resources. After the devastation of Europe in World War II, many former colonial territories, such as India, Kenya, and Indonesia, declared their independence. However, political independence did not necessarily bring economic independence.

The notion of neocolonialism emerged after World War II to better conceptualize the ongoing dependence of newly independent countries on former colonial centers. Kwame Nkrumah (2002, 5), the first president of newly independent Ghana, said that neocolonialism is "based upon the principle of breaking up former large united colonial territories into a number of small non-viable States which are incapable of independent development and must rely upon the former imperial power for defense and even internal security. Their economic and financial systems are linked, as in colonial days, with those of the former colonial ruler." The independence movement of the mid-twentieth century attained the goal of political autonomy in much of the formerly colonized world but not economic self-determination. European colonization, in Guyanese scholar Walter Rodney's (1973) words, underdeveloped Africa. This underdevelopment has fueled exploitative economic relations, devastated environments, disrupted communities, and caused large flows of refugees fleeing for survival. The complex legacy of the Doctrine of Discovery lives on, mutates, and transforms in changing socioeconomic conditions.

At the turn of the twenty-first century, neoliberalism has emerged as the dominant ideological form of the global extractive economy, which David Harvey (2005, 2) defines as "a theory of political economic practices that proposes that human well-being can best be advanced by liberating entrepreneurial freedoms and skills within an institutional framework characterized by strong private property rights, free markets, and free trade." Neoliberalism uses the state to deconstruct institutional arrangements, such as the social safety net, which have served to protect citizens – creating a sense of shock, crisis, and insecurity. When state services and staffing are shrunk, the government becomes less able to cope with demands and more likely to be viewed by the populace as ineffective, if not useless. The push to privatize everything from water treatment to prisons to schools to electronic benefit services actually transfers wealth from the state into the hands of the global financial elite, as the private sector is portrayed as a more efficient service provider than the government. In Kansas, for example, child welfare services began to be privatized in 1997 following some high-profile cases of abuse and neglect. The results of this shift have been mixed indicating many contractual and financial difficulties and a failure to stem the tide of children entering the system (Unruh and Hodgkin, 2004). The Kansas experiment shows that privatization without increased financing, more workers, and better coordination does not solve seemingly intractable problems. Further, privatization reflects a shift from the collective responsibility of government of the people to governance by corporations of the dependent (McDonald, 2014, 66).

The terms *settler colonialism, imperialism, neocolonialism,* and *neoliberalism* describe distinct moments and social formations in the history of the capitalist extractive economy, yet they share similar techniques of control and domination. As slavery was used to control the bodies of Africans to produce wealth for Southern planter society, the mass incarceration of African Americans today can be viewed as a boon both to the private prison industry and to corporations that utilize vastly underpaid prison labor. As biological warfare was used against Indigenous Peoples by settler colonizers who distributed smallpox-laden blankets to cause epidemics the many contemporary health issues of Indigenous Peoples such as diabetes, heart disease, alcoholism, and high rates of COVID-19 mortality can be viewed as the consequences of living in conditions controlled by settler colonialism. As eviction was used as a means to dispossess the native Irish from their traditional lands by colonial English landlords, the same technique is used to push low-income people out of their city neighborhoods and onto the street as global gentrifiers gobble up housing stock in urban centers. Police violence, living in a perpetual state of exception due to the threat of terrorism, gentrification, asymmetrical warfare, and the reckless construction of pipelines and fracking are all contemporary manifestations of colonizing methods of control that disperse and destroy resistance by the public. So, when President Donald Trump pays homage to President Andrew Jackson, it is a gesture of recognition and affirmation of the legacy of settler colonialism, which lives on in manifold ways today.

Trauma studies

Atrocities, as physician Judith Herman (2015) observes, are phenomena that we want to bury and deny as unimaginable in the moral order of the universe. Our response to atrocities often burrows in the netherworld of not knowing or refusing to see. There is, as psychologist Stanley Cohen (2001) points out, a spectrum between knowing and not knowing that ranges from ignorance of facts to refusal to believe the reality to minimizing to outright apathy. When trauma is a collective experience and is denied by the dominant narrative of national identity, then reconciliation and healing become even more difficult, if not impossible. As Judith Herman notes, "the more powerful the perpetrator, the greater is his prerogative to name and define reality, and the more completely his arguments prevail" (2015, 7).

In 2007, for example, the United Nations adopted the Declaration on the Rights of Indigenous Peoples after over twenty years of advocacy by Native leaders. This was an important achievement – to force international attention on the gruesome legacy of settler colonialism that lived on through the contemporary conditions of Indigenous Peoples around the world. Nonetheless, four of the main settler colonial nations (Australia, Canada, New Zealand, and the United States) would only lend support to the declaration if it would have no legally binding measures.

The trauma of colonization has not been collectively recognized by settler nations, despite various attempts at apology and reconciliation (McGonegal, 2009). Reconciliation is a complex societal process that requires a real recognition of the harms and violence committed and an urgency to make right the egregious situation, often through reparations, which offer a concrete means to rectify unjust historical legacies (Cohen, 2001). Reconciliation requires a community that affirms both the humanity and suffering of the victim and undertakes concrete actions to correct old wrongs collectively (Herman, 2015, 8). Remedies and reparations are highly contested issues because they challenge the current social order and the privilege that some may enjoy. This is why narratives of history are key to instilling an understanding of why things are the way they are.

In California, it is still required that fourth-grade pupils do a 'mission project' in which they study the role of Spanish Franciscans in changing the basis of California's economy from hunter-gatherer to agricultural through the establishment of a religious outpost system. Per state educational standards, students make models of the missions and visit sites, but rarely are they told of the brutal treatment of Indigenous Peoples by the friars. In 2015, Pope Francis canonized Father Junipero Serra, against the protests of several groups of Indigenous Californians. Serra initiated the founding of twenty-one missions in present-day California that were designed to convert natives to the Catholic faith. Natives that were converted were kept separate from those who had not accepted Christianity, and some missions flogged and imprisoned those who tried to leave. Many who left were hunted down like fugitive slaves. In an interview on her opposition to the canonization of Father Serra, Professor Deborah Miranda, a literature professor at Washington and Lee University in Virginia and a member of the Ohlone Costanoan Esselen Nation of California, stated that "the missions ended up killing about 90% of the California Indians present at the time of missionization, creating all kinds of cultural and emotional baggage that we still carry to this day. It's about making sure that the truth is heard and that injustices are not continued on into the 21st century" (Burke, 2015).

As the Indigenous of California are often portrayed as a historical and vanquished people, many students often mistakenly assume that the natives of California have long vanished. Indigenous children attend California schools, but their ancestors' story is being told through the lens of the oppressors. How must they feel, to be viewed as an extinct species? The facts of genocide, land theft, and the elimination of the native inevitably give way to distortions in historical representation. Trauma trails persist through generations, as Indigenous Studies scholar Judy Atkinson points out (Atkinson, 2002). How do we understand ourselves and our traumas if we are erased, excluded, and stigmatized? And how can we talk about reconciliation when we are not recognized in all of the complexity of our historical experience?

The recognition and study of intergenerational trauma in the human sciences began in the 1960s, when Western clinicians noticed an alarming rise in the number of children of extermination camp survivors coming in for psychological counseling (Danieli, 2010, 3). The 1960s and 1970s saw a greater number of studies on the impact of the Holocaust on survivors and their children who struggled with anxiety and depression. Many practitioners felt ambivalent, however, about assigning a diagnosis to the suffering of Holocaust survivors and their children. They felt that diagnosing people with trauma due to the Holocaust was dehumanizing because it objectified survivors as victims in need of treatment (Kellermann, 1999). The extremity of the suffering and anguish embodied in the experience of the Nazi genocide was also viewed as beyond the capacity of others to understand. By 1980, there was a diagnosis ("survivor syndrome") in the *Diagnostic and Statistical Manual of Mental Disorders (DSM-III)*, and a burgeoning field of study had developed on the impact of war and genocide trauma on survivors and their children (Danieli, 2010, 3–4).

Research on Holocaust survivors may have represented the first scientific recognition of the impact of intergenerational trauma, but by the late twentieth century, some scholars began to recognize settler colonialism as a form of genocide (e.g., Jaimes, 1992; Legters, 1988; Zinn, 2015). However, it was Indigenous scholars such as Judy Atkinson (2002), Maria Yellow Horse Brave Heart (2003), Bonnie and Eduardo Duran (1995), and Waziyatawin and Michael Yellow Bird (2012) who drew clear lines between the history of settler colonial genocide and current disparities in social, mental, and physical well-being among Indigenous Peoples throughout the world. Using the concept of historical unresolved trauma, Brave Heart, for example, contextualized the Wounded Knee massacre, which killed hundreds, in light of the 1881 government ban on traditional burials, Lakota spirit keeping, and "the wiping of the tears" (Brave Heart and De Bruyn, 1998) Subsequent assimilationist policies such as language and cultural dress bans, boarding schools, displacement from stolen lands, and punitive child protection practices further enforced an alienation of future generations from traditional ways of being and healing. Brave Heart (2003) has argued that the contemporary epidemic of alcoholism, drug abuse, intimate partner violence, and suicide in Indigenous communities globally has roots in the historical trauma and unresolved grief of settler colonial genocide. A social work response must "articulate, conceptualize, and operationalize the need for justice and truth" on behalf of Indigenous Peoples rather than simply ameliorate, empower, or treat (Gray, Coates, and Yellow Bird, 2008, 49).

At the turn of the millennium, emerging research on intergenerational trauma explored the multigenerational impact of various tragedies such as the Armenian genocide (Mangassarian, 2016), African slavery in the United States (Graff, 2014), the round-up of Japanese-Americans into concentration camps during World War II (Nagata, Kim, and Nguyen, 2015), and the Khmer Rouge genocide in Cambodia (Field, Muong, and Sochanvimean, 2013). Internationally, research on the trauma of refugees (Sangalang and Vang, 2017) and endemic intragroup conflict (Fargas-Malet and Dillenburger, 2016) also raised questions about the deep roots of trauma in the colonial past. These scholarly examinations coincided with Truth and Reconciliation Commissions in Guatemala, Chile, and South Africa, which sought to untangle the complex web of civil violence to document human rights violations and make recommendations to enhance societal reconciliation. Australia and Canada also launched commissions to uncover the truth about the impact of settler colonialism on Indigenous communities and explore ways of remediation. Even within non-settler nations, issues of truth and reconciliation have been highly relevant. There has recently been a project in Finland to document the atrocities of the vicious 1918 Civil War in an attempt to clarify the facts of history without the interference of narratives imposed by the victors or vanquished (Kantola, 2014).

To expand the conversation on the textual, visual, historical, cultural, and emotional impact of trauma, an interdisciplinary scholarly field emerged. Literary studies engaged with the legacy of trauma by examining how literature can disrupt the dominant national stories of ourselves, reflecting how historical and social contexts drive memory and forgetting (Caruth, 1996; LaCapra, 2016; Schacter and Coyle, 1995). At the same time, cultural trauma theory was viewed as inadequate by many postcolonial literary scholars because of its Eurocentric orientation and affirmation of stasis and melancholia as appropriate responses to trauma (Visser, 2011, 270). Others have pointed out that trauma studies still largely focuses on a Euro-American context, privileging the experiences of white Europeans while neglecting non-Western and minority cultural traumas (Andermahr, 2015, 500). These critical scholars have challenged the Eurocentric bias of Western traumatic histories, arguing that they must be seen as entangled with histories of colonial trauma (Craps and Buelens, 2008).

By the late 1990s, many began to challenge the notion of the uniqueness of the trauma of the Shoah (or the Nazi Holocaust of the Jews) by extending the notion of genocide to settler colonialism. David Moshman (2001) argues that the Eurocentric conceptualization of the Holocaust as unique and unmatched in world history tends to render the other major genocides such as that of Indigenous Peoples, Armenians, Cambodians, and Rwandans invisible. Rather than minimizing the suffering of European Jews, Moshman seeks to better delineate the societal processes that lead to these horrendous historical events and to break out of the restrictive conceptual structures that prevent us from being conscious of other atrocities and thus acting to recognize and remedy, as well as prevent. In *The Abu Gharib Effect* (2007), historian Stephen Eisenman reflects on a similar process with the public indifference that accompanied published images of the torture of Iraqis by American soldiers arguing that there is a colonial aesthetic tradition of sanctioning the death and torture of non-Europeans and animals. When victims are seen as less than human, then atrocities are minimized. As noted earlier, Indigenous scholars such as Maria Yellow Horse Brave Heart (2003) and Bonnie and Eduardo Duran (1995) have challenged the Eurocentrism of emerging trauma studies by applying the framework of "genocide survival" to the continuing suffering of Indigenous Peoples. Trauma studies is, after all, fundamentally about the future in the sense that it seeks to build a bridge between the incomprehensibility of past horrific events and ways that we can collectively move forward through recognition of historic wrongs and by enacting just remedies (Ramadanovic, 1998).

Knowing the past requires an openness to uncovering factual history and a willingness to engage with self-deception and the societal minimization of trauma. Societal recognition demands a readiness to listen to the experiences of others, particularly marginalized communities whose stories have been silenced. In short: "The systematic study of psychological trauma . . . depends on the support of a political movement. Indeed, whether such study can be pursued or discussed in public is itself a political question," according to Judith Herman (2015, 9–10).

The trauma of settler colonialism exists not just in the genocide, dispossession, enslavement, exile, segregation, mass incarceration, and trafficking of Indigenous and other colonized peoples but also (and perhaps most insidiously) in the internally imposed ideologies of domination that stretch down through many generations (Fanon, 1963). Judy Atkinson (2002, 258) has pointed out that colonization makes, names, and labels oppressed people as lesser and Other, which reinforces separation and fragmentation resulting in people feeling devalued, excluded, and lost. The aim of settler schools, media, and many other social formations is to colonize the minds of the populace because these institutions are deeply intertwined with the material extractive capitalist structures of nations. Explicit settler ideologies and values are inculcated in both oppressors and the oppressed through a colonization of the mind (Memmi, 2016). This cognitive process utilizes coercion and persuasion to internalize settler colonial ways of being, knowing, and acting by diminishing or excluding other ways of knowing as false, lesser, or backwards.

Historical trauma has been defined as cumulative and collective trauma that produces psychological and emotional suffering in individuals and communities. Historical unresolved grief can emerge in the wake of historical trauma due to multiple, rapid community losses through genocide, land theft, and cultural erasure. The inability to mourn and manage grief in culturally and spiritually appropriate ways due to the suppression of Indigenous practices can intensify the sense of unresolved grief (Brave Heart and De Bruyn, 1998). Suicide, substance abuse, and depression, all symptoms of complicated and unresolved grief, are often prevalent in communities with historical trauma. Communities subject to settler colonialism have nonetheless shown remarkable resilience in the face of historical trauma. As Brave Heart and De Bruyn (1998) has pointed out, it is important to make a distinction between historical trauma and historical trauma response, in which people can manifest great strength, resistance, and courage despite the weight of oppression and unresolved grief. Recent demonstrations in the United States protesting the violence of the police, an institution which has roots in slave patrols and segregation, shows how people with historical trauma have the resilience to resist despite ongoing oppression.

Brazilian educator Paulo Freire wrote about the need to challenge the colonization of the mind through the process of conscientization, which he defined as raising critical awareness of one's social reality through reflection and action (Freire, 2000). Conscientization challenges the individual and collective alienation from the self and culture imposed by settler colonial masters and provides an avenue for resistance and social change. The spark of decolonizing the mind thus comes from the steel of conscientization, struck by the flint of memory work.

The importance of memory work

Our sense of identity, belonging, and social order is intertwined with group narratives of social memory that command powerful emotional authority. The anthropologist Benedict Anderson (2006) once described modern nation-states as "imagined communities" because they bind large groups of people together through a narrative leap of collective storytelling. Nationalism is both a narrative and an ideology that unites people and often enforces the boundaries between us and them. It also reflects a sense of kinship across and beyond borders in which people proclaim a common story of origin based on a shared place, culture, and social memory. This imagined national identity, however, is woven of selective histories and perspectives that often exclude those considered to be outsiders, even if those seen as strangers are members of the national body politic.

The profession of social work emerged with the modern nation-state as an activity legitimated by the state and aimed at mitigating some of the worst impacts of extractive capitalism. Social work is framed by national policies that aim to enhance greater social cohesion and are implemented through evidence-based practices that often pay little notice to the concerns, ways of knowing, and needs of diverse communities. As a social change and human rights profession, social work is obligated to advocate for the most marginalized and vulnerable in society. Poverty, dispossession, and disadvantage emerge from a context of social inequality and oppression that has deep roots in historical injustice and trauma. *Memory work* signifies the process of exploring the past through complex personal and collective memories situated in space and time through diverse experiences, as well as cultural and political artifacts (Fraser and Mitchell, 2015). Memory work, however, is rarely considered an appropriate or evidence-based intervention for healing.

Settler colonialism is built upon the conscious forgetting of Indigenous Peoples' histories, cultures, and ways of being. This social amnesia obscures the invasions, slavery, policing, and genocides that have enforced the subjugation and oppression of Indigenous Peoples by settler colonists. As West Indian poet Derek Walcott (2006, 370) noted, "Amnesia is the true history of the New World." In the United States, forgetting is crucial for the maintenance of systems of oppression because it preserves national myths of egalitarianism, exceptionalism, and fairness obscuring systemic histories of racism, sexism, ableism, and homophobia. Social memory plays both public and collective as well as personal and individual roles (Galanter, 2002, 5). Memory work, therefore, is key to challenging and overturning systems of oppression and finding ways to heal and liberate oneself from the pall of colonial ideologies by supporting healthy identity development.

Paul Connerton (2008, 59) writes of different types of forgetting and notes that "forgetting is not a unitary phenomenon." Repressive erasure, for instance, seeks to deny uncomfortable historical facts that may challenge current constructions of identity. Censorship and the removal of images from historical photographs under Stalin is one example of how a state attempted to reshape social memory through erasure. There are many statues of Confederate military leaders in localities throughout the southern part of the United States – generals John C. Breckenridge, Robert E. Lee, and John Hunt Morgan, among others – that were erected long after the American Civil War as monuments to prevailing white supremacy, while the first memorial to the victims of the trans-Atlantic slave trade in the United States was only unveiled in the grounds of the United Nations in New York City in 2015. The recent removal of Confederate statues in the South, sometimes in the dead of night by masked city workers due to threats of violence and sometimes through mass resistance to authorities, demonstrates the visceral investment that many have in narratives of social memory that distort and repress historical fact.

Repressive erasure is often state directed because it seeks to deny historical memory that may challenge the current social order. There is also forgetting that is constitutive of a new identity, meaning that some elements of historical fact may be repressed because they are incompatible with emerging national narratives of identity. The independence of India as a unified national identity after the fall of the British Raj can be seen as one example of the construction of a new identity from a multiplicity of diverse ethnic identities. Forgetting, in this sense, is viewed as less important than the birth of a new narrative of commonality and mutuality. Finally, there is structural amnesia, which fabricates a system that encourages certain types of social memory while leaving no room for other types of memory. As Connerton (2008) points out, the prevalent use of patrilineal genealogy in British peerage rendered matrilineal lines tangential to the determination of origin and rights. The practice of suppressing and diminishing the memory of matrilineal lines thus reinforced male dominance in society. Repressing or forgetting certain facts or narratives contrary to the dominant account of origin reinforces a certain type of identity and social memory that strengthens particular views of the present and visions of the future. Yet repressed memory does not dissipate and will continue to haunt communities and contribute to the cycle of intergenerational trauma. Societies run the risk of repeating atrocities and abuses by failing to remember and learn from the roles and responsibilities of perpetrators and bystanders. The manifold consequences of colonization psychically, socially, and materially still shroud many communities making forgiveness and reconciliation elusive when memory work remains incomplete.

In the opening lines of *The Faraway Nearby*, Rebecca Solnit (2014, 3) wrote that stories are "our compasses and architecture; we navigate by them, we build our sanctuaries and prisons out of them and to be without a story is to be lost in the vastness of a world that spreads in all directions like arctic tundra or sea ice." Stories are born of the memory of experience and trace a shifting geography of self, community, and place. Decolonizing memory work activates the repressed past and layers different time periods in relation to the present and future. It opens up how we learn to know and understand ourselves through the matrix of power and oppression. It ponders how we should transmit and understand the entanglements of the traumatic past. Memory work militates against what writer Chimamanda Adichie calls "the danger of a single story" (Adichie, 2009). By recovering our own voices and unique stories, memory work confronts dominant and silencing perspectives by opening up a space for the stories of the marginalized and voiceless. It recognizes the coexistence of multiple histories and memories and considers how deeply social memory and forgetting is intertwined. In acknowledging the limitations of official history, memory work also considers the problematics of forgetting and overlooking. Just as decolonized remembering involves challenging the epistemology of official maps and histories of culture and events, memory work demands contemporary political consciousness and direct action.

Memory work confronts violent trauma and the haunting that generations of repression, silence, and disempowerment has produced. It engages with the real pain that the trauma of history has caused. In *Trauma Trails, Recreating Song Lines*, Judy Atkinson (2002) discussed a program called We Al-li, which she facilitated with people deeply enmeshed in individual and collective trauma. Of Jima, Budjalung, and Celtic-German heritage herself, she pointed out the multiple layers of loss Indigenous Peoples dealt with including the destruction of traditional knowledge, ceremonies, and relationship to land and people had transgenerational impact. Maria Yellow Horse Brave Heart (1998) wrote about the Return to the Sacred Path, a psychosocial intervention and trauma resolution process aimed at human services professionals working with the Lakota. In naming and processing a reality that has often been obscured, memory work heals through remembering, recognizing, reimagining, and dreaming new futurities.

References

Adichie, C. N. (2009). *TEDTalks: Chimamanda Adichie – The Danger of a Single Story*. New York, N.Y.: Films Media Group.

Agamben, G. 2012. State of Exception. *Phainomena*, 21(1): 63–172.

Andermahr, S. 2015. Decolonizing Trauma Studies: Trauma and Postcolonialism – Introduction. *Humanities*, 2015(4): 500–505.

Anderson, B. 2006. *Imagined Communities: Reflections on the Origin and Spread of Nationalism*. Rev. ed. New York: Verso.

Anderson, D. G. 2000. *Identity and Ecology in Arctic Siberia: The Number One Reindeer Brigade*. Oxford: Oxford University Press.

Andrea, A., and Neel, C. 2011. Moving Sugar Plantation Laborers to the Atlantic Islands. In *World History Encyclopedia*. Santa Barbara, CA: ABC-Clio.

Atkinson, J. 2002. *Trauma Trails, Recreating Song Lines*. North Melbourne: Spinifex.

Berkey, C. 2005. City of Sherrill v. Oneida Indian Nation. *American Indian Law Review*, 30(2): 373–384.

Brave Heart, M. Y. H. 2003. The Historical Trauma Response among Natives and Its Relationship with Substance Abuse: A Lakota Illustration. *Journal of Psychoactive Drugs*, 35(1): 7–13.

Brave Heart, M. Y. H., and DeBruyn, L. 1998. The American Indian Holocaust: Healing Historical Unresolved Grief. *American Indian and Alaska Native Mental Health Research*, 8(2): 60–82.

Briere, J., and Spinazzola, J. 2005. Phenomenology and Psychological Assessment of Complex Posttraumatic States. *Journal of Traumatic Stress*, 18(5): 401–412.

Burke, D. 2015. Pope Francis Canonizes Controversial Saint Serra. *CNN*. Accessed 14 February 2019 at www.cnn.com/2015/09/23/us/pope-junipero-serra-canonization/index.html.

Caruth, C. 1996. *Unclaimed Experience: Trauma, Narrative, and History*. Baltimore: Johns Hopkins University Press.

Chamovitz, D. 2017. *What a Plant Knows: A Field Guide to the Senses*. New York: Farrar, Straus and Giroux.

Cohen, S. 2001. *States of Denial: Knowing About Atrocities and Suffering*. Cambridge: Polity.

Connerton, P. 2008. *How Societies Remember*. Cambridge: Cambridge University Press.

Craps, S., and Buelens, G. 2008. Introduction: Postcolonial Trauma Novels. *Studies in the Novel*, 40(1–2) (Spring/Summer): 1–12.

Danieli, Y. 2010. *International Handbook of Multigenerational Legacies of Trauma*. New York: Plenum.

Dobyns, H. F., and Swagerty, W. R. 1983. *Their Number Become Thinned: Native American Population Dynamics in Eastern North America*. Knoxville: University of Tennessee Press.

Donnelly, J. 2001. *The Great Irish Potato Famine*. Thrupp, Stroud, Gloucestershire: Sutton.

Dunbar-Ortiz, R. 2009. *Interview*. Accessed 3 April 2019 at www.commondreams.org/newswire/2009/01/28/obama-claims-us-not-born-colonial-power.

Dunbar-Ortiz, R. 2014. *An Indigenous Peoples' History of the United States*. Old Saybrook, CT: Tantor Media.

Duran, E., and Duran, B. 1995. *Native American Postcolonial Psychology*. SUNY Series in Transpersonal and Humanistic Psychology. Albany: State University of New York Press.

Eisenman, S. 2007. *The Abu Gharib Effect*. London: Reaction Books.

Fanon, F. 1963. *The Wretched of the Earth*. New York: Grove Press.

Fargas-Malet, M., and Dillenburger, K. 2016. Intergenerational Transmission of Conflict-Related Trauma in Northern Ireland: A Behavior Analytic Approach. *Journal of Aggression, Maltreatment, and Trauma*, 24(4): 436–454.

Field, N., Muong, S., and Sochanvimean, V. 2013. Parental Styles in the Intergenerational Transmission of Trauma Stemming from the Khmer Rouge Regime in Cambodia. *American Journal of Orthopsychiatry*, 83(4): 483–494.

Fraser, H., and Mitchell, D. 2015. Feminist Memory Work in Action: Method and Practicalities. *Qualitative Social Work*, 14(3): 321–337.

Freire, P. 2000. *Pedagogy of the Oppressed*. New York: Bloomsbury.

Galanter, M. 2002. Righting Old Wrongs. In *Breaking the Cycles of Hatred: Memory, Law, and Repair*, edited by M. Minow and N. Rosenblum, 107–131. Princeton, NJ: Princeton University Press.

Gilgoff, D. 2009. "Barack Obama Grants First TV Interview as President to Arabic Network." *US News*. Accessed 5 March 2019 at www.usnews.com/news/blogs/god-and-country/2009/01/27/barack-obama-grants-first-tv-interview-as-president-to-arabic-network.

Graff, G. 2014. The Intergenerational Trauma of Slavery and Its Aftermath. *Journal of Psychohistory*, 41(3) (Winter): 181–197.

Gray, M., Coates, J., and Yellow Bird, M. (eds.). 2008. *Indigenous Social Work Around the World: Towards Culturally Relevant Education and Practice*. Aldershot: Ashgate.

Gray, M., Coates, J., Yellow Bird, M., and Hetherington, T. (eds.). 2016. *Decolonizing Social Work*. London: Routledge.

Haines, R., McDonald, J., and Shlomowitz, R. 2001. Mortality and Voyage Length in the Middle Passage Revisited. *Explorations in Economic History*, 38: 503–533.

Harvey, D. 2005. *A Brief History of Neoliberalism*. Oxford: Oxford University Press.

Herman, J. L. 2015. *Trauma and Recovery*. New York: Basic Books.

Igler, D. 2017. *Great Ocean – Pacific Worlds from Captain Cook to the Gold Rush*. Oxford: Oxford University Press.

Ingold, T. 2000. *The Perception of the Environment: Essays on Livelihood, Dwelling and Skill*. London: Routledge.

Jaimes, M. 1992. *The State of Native America: Genocide, Colonization, and Resistance*. Race and Resistance. Boston: South End.

Kantola, A. 2014. The Therapeutic Imaginary in Memory Work: Mediating the Finnish Civil War in Tampere. *Memory Studies*, 7(1) (January): 92–107.

Kellermann, N. P. F. 1999. Diagnosis of Holocaust Survivors and Their Children. *Israel Journal of Psychiatry*, 36(1): 55–65.

Kramer, J. 2016. (Re)mapping Terra Nullius: Hindmarsh, Wik and Native Title Legislation in Australia. *International Journal for the Semiotics of Law/Revue Internationale De Sémiotique Juridique*, 29(1) (March): 191–212.

Lacapra, D. 2016. Trauma, History, Memory, Identity: What Remains? *History and Theory*, 55(3) (October): 375–400.

Legters, L. 1988. The American Genocide. *Policy Studies Journal*, 16(4) (June): 768–677.

Loewen, J. W. 2018. *Lies My Teacher Told Me: Everything Your American History Textbook Got Wrong*. New York: The New Press.

Long March to Rome. 2016. *The Long March to Rome*. Accessed 23 March 2019 at https://longmarchtorome.com/the-creator-has-been-heard/

Mangassarian, S. 2016. 100 Years of Trauma: The Armenian Genocide and Intergenerational Cultural Trauma. *Journal of Aggression, Maltreatment & Trauma*, 25(4): 371–381.

McDonald, C. 2014. *Challenging Social Work: The Institutional Context of Practice*. Basingstoke: Palgrave Macmillan.

McGonegal, J. 2009. *Imagining Justice: The Politics of Postcolonial Forgiveness and Reconciliation*. Montreal: McGill-Queen's University Press.

McGregor, K. E. 2012. Time, Memory and Historical Justice: An Introduction. *Time & Society*, 21(1): 5–20.

McKenna, E., and Pratt, S. L. 2015. *American Philosophy: From Wounded Knee to the Present*. New York: Bloomsbury.

Memmi, A. 2016. *The Colonizer and the Colonized*. Boston: Beacon Press.

Miller, R. J., Ruru, J., Behrendt, L., and Lindberg, T. 2014. *Discovering Indigenous Lands: The Doctrine of Discovery in the English Colonies*. Oxford: Oxford University Press.

Mintz, S. 2019. *Childhood and Transatlantic Slavery*. Case study 57, Children and Youth in History. Accessed at https://chnm.gmu.edu/cyh/case-studies/57.

Mokyr, J., and Grda, C. 2002. What Do People Die of During Famines: The Great Irish Famine in Comparative Perspective. *European Review of Economic History*, 6(3) (December): 339–363.

Moshman, D. 2001. Conceptual Constraints on Thinking about Genocide. *Journal of Genocide Research*, 3(3) (August): 431–450.

Nagata, D., Kim, J., and Nguyen, T. 2015. Processing Cultural Trauma: Intergenerational Effects of the Japanese American Incarceration. *Journal of Social Issues*, 71(2) (June): 356–370.

Njoh, A. 2017. Toponymic Inscription as an Instrument of Power in Africa: The Case of Colonial and Post-colonial Dakar and Nairobi. *Journal of Asian and African Studies*, 52(8): 1174–1192.

Nkrumah, K. 2002. *Neo-colonialism: The Last Stage of Imperialism*. London: Panaf.

Ramadanovic, P. 1998. Unclaimed Experience: Trauma, Narrative, and History. *Diacritics*, 28(4) (Winter): 54–67.

Reséndez, A. 2017. *The Other Slavery: The Uncovered Story of Indian Enslavement in America*. Boston: Mariner Books.

Rodney, W. 1973. *How Europe Underdeveloped Africa*. Washington, DC: Howard University Press.

Said, E. 1993. *Culture and Imperialism*. London: Chatto & Windus.

Sangalang, C., and Vang, C. 2017. Intergenerational Trauma in Refugee Families: A Systematic Review. *Journal of Immigrant and Minority Health*, 19(3) (June): 745–754.

Schacter, D., and Coyle, J. 1995. *Memory Distortion: How Minds, Brains, and Societies Reconstruct the Past*. Cambridge, MA: Harvard University Press.

Solnit, R. 2014. *The Faraway Nearby*. London: Granta Books.

Stannard, D. E. 1992. *American Holocaust: Columbus and the Conquest of the New World*. New York: Oxford University Press.

Unruh, J. K., and Hodgkin, D. 2004. The Role of Contract Design in Privatization of Child Welfare Services: The Kansas Experience. *Children and Youth Services Review*, 26(8): 771–783.

Visser, I. 2011. Trauma Theory and Postcolonial Literary Studies. *Journal of Postcolonial Writing*, 47(3): 270–282.

Walcott, D. 2006. "The Muse of History." In *The Post-colonial Studies Reader*. 2nd ed., edited by Bill Ashcroft, Gareth Griffiths, and Helen Tiffin, 370–374. London: Routledge.

Watson, B. 2012. *Buying America from the Indians: Johnson v. McIntosh and the History of Native Land Rights*. Norman: University of Oklahoma Press.

Waziyatawin, and Yellow Bird, M. (eds.). 2012. *For Indigenous Minds Only: A Decolonization Handbook*. School of American Research. Santa Fe, NM: Santa Fe Press.

Weisbord, R. 2003. The King, the Cardinal and the Pope: Leopold II's Genocide in the Congo and the Vatican. *Journal of Genocide Research*, 5(1): 35–45.

Yellow Bird, M. 1999. Indian, American Indian, and Native Americas: Counterfeit Identities. *Winds of Change: A Magazine for American Indian Education and Opportunity*, 14: 1.

Zinn, H. 2015. *A People's History of the United States*. New York: Harper Perennial Modern Classics. Reprint.

3 Confronting professional imperialism and moving towards integrative healing

KRIS SHARES A STORY

On a sunny April morning in 2018, approximately thirty Fresno State under-graduate social work students marched out of the Professional Human Services building at California State University and began chanting: "Student power!" The culturally and ethnically diverse group carried colorful signs reading: "Let's talk," "The DSWE [Department of Social Work Education] needs transparency," and "Don't call me unqualified, qualify me!" Latinx, Hmong, African American, and Euro American undergraduate students rallied together to express their bitter disappointment at the results of the admissions process for their university's master's program in social work. After the decisions had been rendered the previous week, rumors swirled down the hallways suggesting that Fresno State professors did not find their own students qualified enough for the graduate program. Students compared notes on their applications and grew increasingly perturbed about the lack of departmental transparency and clarity about their perceptions of widely disparate scores and results. They began to ask about how the requirements for the applications were constructed and why. They wondered aloud how so few Hmong, Native American, and African American students appeared to gain admission into the program. Students questioned how the department devised criteria to assess who would make good potential social workers for this culturally diverse and impoverished region.

California State University, Fresno has a student body that is about half Latinx, 17% Euro American, 6% South East Asian, and the remainder divided amongst African American, international students, and a variety of other identities. The typical Fresno State social work student does not fit into the stereotype of an undergraduate college student living in a dormitory with generous parental financial support. Most Fresno State students encounter multiple barriers as they proceed along their degree path. They are often first-generation university students; they hold down several jobs to survive and support families while studying and interning; they commute long distances from small rural towns; and they write complex academic papers in English as a second language on the foundation of an underperforming high school education. Fresno State students represent the wide cultural and ethnic diversity of the Central Valley and have roots in Indigenous genocide as well as Southeast Asian, Latino, Armenian, Dust Bowl, and African American diasporas of agricultural workers who have survived and thrived in this roughhewn and socially conservative locale. Many students have had difficult experiences with immigration raids, poverty, discrimination, substance misuse, trauma, parents absent due to crushing work obligations, environmental injustice, and interpersonal violence. These students are not strangers to the issues and communities that engage with social workers.

Social work graduate admissions at Fresno State are constructed similarly to many other settler colonial universities. The process and criteria for admissions employ a grammar of detached professionalism that forces students to prove their competence and ability to perform in the colonized curriculum. Based on four main criteria – grades in undergraduate studies, the personal statement, paid working experience, and the score on a costly standardized exam – a committee confidentially ranks applicants and renders decisions. However, as students did further research on admissions, they began to question whether the settler colonial process that defined these benchmarks privileged certain groups over others due to the weight placed on evidence that required money. The Graduate Record Examination (GRE), for example, is a standardized test intended to predict who will succeed in graduate studies. However, some studies indicate that the GRE is a better measure of socioeconomic status, race, and gender rather than of perseverance and resilience in pursuing a graduate degree (Clayton, 2016). The test itself runs about 200 dollars, and many students take it multiple times. Preparation courses for the GRE can run from 1,000 to 3,000 dollars.

Avelina Charles, who was close to completing her bachelor's degree in social work at Fresno State, informed her advisor that she was not going to apply for the master's in social work program. "I told him the one and only reason why I would not apply at Fresno State," said Avelina. "I let him know that the mandatory GRE was not made for people like me. I told him that I am Chicana, I come from a low socioeconomic background, and I have a learning disability. That would be three barriers already before applying."

Students also asked why their year-long undergraduate social work internships did not count as work experience. What use, they felt, were the many hours they spent in supervised social work training, if it counted for nothing? Students wondered how personal statements were read and assessed: they insisted on greater transparency from the department to explain how these criteria were applied to students from diverse cultural, ethnic, and social groups. They wanted demographic data to better measure how inclusive the department admissions process actually was.

When social work students James Borunda, Avelina Charles, and Rosa Salmeron took up a bullhorn and led students on the walkout, they rallied in front of the windows where the department was holding a faculty meeting. At the start of the meeting, someone closed the blinds so that students could not see in and faculty could not see out. The meeting was called to order, and the hullabaloo outside was ignored. Students then decided to walk into the faculty meeting and surrounded the people sitting at the conference table chanting "student power" and waving their placards. The meeting chair told students that they were not on the agenda and had to leave. They were advised to go through proper channels to request a spot on the agenda in the meeting after two weeks. The students retreated, and the opportunity for open dialogue vanished as each side regrouped and planned their strategy.

James, Rosa, and Avelina met with the department chair to discuss the dispute. Rosa said: "The chair said that we didn't have a dog in the fight. James got into the program; Avelina didn't apply and was admitted somewhere else; and I didn't apply to any master's program because I was going into the Peace Corps. She didn't understand what our driving force was and why we wouldn't drop it." When students later met with deans and administrators, they felt reprimanded for criticizing the department. Administrators asked: "Did you learn anything from this experience, so that next time you could do things differently? Do you think you might have overreacted with the actions you took?" Students felt frustrated and diminished as none of their concerns about equity and social justice in the program were addressed.

When students finally were able to get on the agenda and attend the faculty meeting after two weeks, they entered a packed room of academics both grim-faced and curious. A student reporter from the university newspaper was told to leave by the dean of the college, though the Fresno State communications officer was present, keenly following the discussion. Students were informed that they needed to follow the chain of command to register complaints or queries. Making noise with walkouts and protests was not the way to ask questions, several members of the assembled faculty said. They were assured the admissions process was fair but were still not given detailed answers to their questions. The students were not satisfied after the faculty meeting and continued their protests demanding transparency and more discussion.

Communication between the administration, faculty, and student activists was framed in top-down neutral professionalism because the only ways and means of discussing were defined by faculty schedules and rules of order which increased the power of the administration and faculty over students. The use of an Indigenous communication tool such as the talking stick, in which each participant has an equal opportunity to speak, could have provided an opportunity to reduce the hierarchy of voices, open up silence, and enhance connection with all of the parties involved. Such a technique could have provided a creative platform to engage with one another to create a new vision of the purpose and goals of the social work program. By remaining within the comfort of the neutral professional paradigm, however, the institutional actors missed the chance for transformative dialogue and resolution.

Students, administration, and faculty were at a loggerheads reflecting the distinct ways of understanding the core mission of social work and how it should be practiced. Students, who had completed undergraduate studies in the field, saw social work as a calling to activist social justice organizing: "Be the change you want to see," read their banners. However, the administrative response was that they should not question decisions, especially not by waving signs and chanting.

Change, in the institution's view, came through meetings at which the evolution of structures, policies, and processes was discussed. These meetings were generally restricted to institutional actors, excluding community and students. Indeed, many of the administration and faculty felt that the social work program should concern itself with educating students realistically for the job market as therapists, counselors, program administrators, and child protection workers, not promoting a tradition of loud protests which would never lead to a job. So, how do we reconcile these different emphases in social work as a discipline, community action, and profession? What is the core mission of social work after all? Social work researcher Leslie Margolin (1997, 3–4) frames it this way:

> The interesting question to me is not why social workers are 'unfaithful' to some original calling, but, rather, why they are so often uncomfortable practicing it. I want to know why social workers are so ready to bail out. But instead of blaming difficult work conditions, inflexible bureaucracy, uncooperative and unappreciative clients. . . . I point the finger at the profession itself – at a tradition that forces social workers into the most debilitating sorts of denial, hypocrisy, and double binds. My take on the matter, then, is that 'the problem' is not that social workers are abandoning the core mission; the problem *is* the core mission.

Questioning the construction of the 'core mission' of social work as professionalized, hierarchical, and bureaucratic requires the recognition of its settler colonial roots. Shifting our view of the mission of social work means becoming aware of the deep ties between social work and the settler colonial state. The Fresno State student protest raised many questions: How do we assess qualifications to become a social worker, and who decides? Are social work programs accountable to the communities in which they operate? Who should gain access to social work educational programs? What are the proper channels to advocate for change? Can 'non-experts' talk back to experts and challenge them to weigh the opinions of community members equally? How do institutions that are explicitly committed to diversity actually enact diversity? How could Fresno State social work education be understood within the Indigenous context of Central California? Stakeholders are often uncomfortable about what challenging settler colonial structures and processes would mean for the university, curriculum, admissions, faculty, and students. But clearly the ideological legacy of settler colonialism continues to thrive in everyday institutional policies and practices.

In the end, the students were denied the right to have access to the demographic information of admissions despite many meetings with administrators. They only received information after a Freedom of Information Act request was made on their behalf by a faculty member, and by that time summer had started, and students had scattered. Some of the information appeared to provide evidence to their perceptions of racial disparities but there were still many questions. Though some of the protesters were eventually accepted into the program through the waiting list, many decided to go elsewhere. Some struggled with the cognitive dissonance between the ideals of advocacy they had learned – and fervently believed in – and the lack of transparency and inclusion that they experienced with the department. Many felt cynical about the whole process. The institution managed to control the discourse, and nothing really changed. James Borunda joined the new class of graduate students in social work at Fresno State and received his master's degree in 2020. He plans to focus on community work. Avelina Charles went to graduate in another master's program. Rosa Salmeron joined the Peace Corps.

Lessons on pathways

The profession of social work, as we discussed in the first chapter, emerged from a settler colonial framework and was constructed on a complex foundation of social reform, individualist helping approaches, modern methods of population control, and community advocacy. These forces have shaped social work's professional identity, practices, and the curriculum it uses to train future professionals. Further, it has defined ways of processing and understanding interaction and discourse. As Fresno State social work students found when they called for common dialogue, social work administration and faculty were enmeshed in systems that privileged closed bureaucratic meetings, top-down perspectives, hierarchies, and insular governance. Dissent was viewed as profoundly threatening to the system. Could the students' protests have offered radical possibilities to administration and faculty to be change makers in the institution? Could shifting the adversarial construction of the admissions dispute towards a conversation potentially have changed the situation, opening up opportunities for dialogue and inclusive program renewal?

Social work as a scientific discipline and practice was born of a quintessentially modernist paradigm. It privileges settler colonial ways of understanding knowledge and acting as experts using boards of accreditation that define, shape, and monitor university-level training for social workers. The process for decision making and discussion in social work generally follows the hierarchical process of Robert's Rules of Order rather than the participatory democracy of the talking stick. As social work professionals, we draw on specialized scientific literature largely hermetically constructed (and sealed behind paywalls) by small groups of experts in Western countries to define scientifically sound concepts of wellness and ways to treat and heal. Research on international social work is dominated by Westerners and their perspectives, often erasing local and Indigenous voices and perpetuating "a paternalistic framing of non-Western cultures, knowledge systems and social care traditions [and] elitism and exclusion" (Haug, 2005). Increasingly, the language of competency and evidence-based practice has privileged technical-bureaucratic ways of understanding social work practice over reflective approaches in an attempt to provide greater risk management and accountability (Wilson, 2013). However, some studies indicate that the growing proceduralization and standardization of practices in areas such as child protection may even lead to greater risk as simply following organizational protocols may not take into account the need for critical thinking in complex and difficult situations

(Broadhurst, Hall, Wastell, White, and Pithouse, 2010). Contemporary language in social work emphasizing narrow definitions of competence and evidence excludes other voices and perspectives as lacking the proper expertise, thus reinforcing systems of dominance and oppression (Fook, 2011).

In the early 1980s, social work professor James Midgely (1981) coined the term "professional imperialism" to describe how social work professionals uncritically transfer settler colonial theories of helping, development, and human rights to formerly colonized countries through international social work models and practices. Though his critique focused on development theories, Midgely (2008) recently pointed out that the same dynamic of unreflective and uncritical imperial professionalism constructs much of the contemporary discourse on international social work. Unless social work engages in memory work, deep structures of settler colonialism will continue to frame much of the project of international social work practice (Haug, 2005). As Payne and Askeland (2008) note, attempts to create global standards for social work practice with common learning materials and the imposition of the use of English as a lingua franca represent some of the ways that local and Indigenous cultures are erased and bypassed as sources of knowledge. Further, these closed systems of international social work discourses are exclusive to those who hold the requisite professional credentials, speak the dominant language, and are affiliated with large institutions.

Being an expert and knowing what to do are seen as the overriding characteristics of the status of a professional, whereas ambiguity, ambivalence, and uncertainty are thought to be signs of an amateur. When a distressed client is referred to a mental health practitioner, for example, we expect a definitive outcome to occur in a timely manner. If there is no change from the unwanted behavior, then we tend to seek out flaws in the therapist or the method utilized or even in the client herself. We debate the merits and shortcomings of the practitioner's methods because we expect science to have a solution to alleviate the suffering of the client.

In training the spotlight on symptoms, we thus often overlook the significance of the broader context of the individual's lifeworld when considering the issue at hand. We exclude the power of historical trauma and role of structural violence as secondary to the diagnosis that is being treated. We often do not recognize how settler values continue to pervade ways that the profession and system views the individual, community, and healing. The narrow focus on intervention and evidence-based skill reinforces a fragmented view of the client as a set of symptoms to treat. Moreover, this approach constructs the human services professional as a modern-day alchemist expected to harness the forces of scientific knowledge to transform distressed and oppressed people into high functioning members of contemporary settler society without fundamentally altering the unjust power relations that often have ignited the dysfunction in the first place.

To return to our story, the students' protest over admissions policies reflects the limitations of settler colonial frameworks of knowing and acting. Administrators and faculty focused on the behaviors of the students (walkouts and protests) and attempted to manage the risk to the institution by using hierarchical methods of controlling discussions and decisions. In this way, the context and point of the student protest was marginalized and rendered unimportant. While social work explicitly underlines the goal of human rights and social justice, in situations like the one in our story, we can see that an imperial professional approach to dealing with oppression and social injustice in fact reaffirms settler colonial domination and exclusion. If they are not preemptively foreclosed, other points of departures and ways of knowing and interacting are imaginable.

In what follows, we briefly outline the contexts of emerging integrative and decolonizing social work practices. We then bring an Indigenous worldview to the center of this discussion about healing and well-being not out of a false nostalgia for an idealized past or with a superficial nod to facile inclusivity but as a fundamental challenge to the intellectual and material legacy of settler colonialism which has caused so much harm. Departing from an Indigenous worldview forces us to consider different ways of being, knowing, and acting in relation to human well-being.

Emerging themes in integrative and decolonizing social work

Decolonization is a major academic framework in Native American/American Indian and Indigenous Studies. It refers to understanding, undoing, and overcoming the myriad negative and disabling effects of colonialism. Colonialism celebrates the ideas, stories, history, beliefs, and values of the colonizer (the oppressor); at the same time, it trivializes, ignores, and subjugates those of the colonized (the oppressed, Indigenous Peoples). Decolonization is a liberatory and interrogatory approach used to critique and act against colonial structures, narratives, and methods. Books such as *Decolonizing Methodologies* by Linda Tuhiwai Smith, *Indigenous Methodologies* by Margaret Kovach (2009); *Environmental Social Work* by Gray, Coates, and Hetherington (2013); *Indigenous Social Work Around the World: Towards Culturally Relevant Education and Practice* by Gray, Coates, and Yellow Bird (2008); and the trailblazing *Decolonizing Social Work* by Gray, Coates, Yellow Bird, and Hetherington (2013) have opened up new ways of theorizing about decolonization in education and social work. Social work is still in the early days of exploring decolonization in its field and considering ways to apply it to social work education and practice.

Integrative social work is a healing-oriented approach that recognizes that the well-being of the entire person depends on the incorporation and balance of three areas: (1) an individual's lifestyle, experience, culture, belief and values systems; (2) the access and interactions one has with human-designed structures, systems and processes; and (3) the access and interactions one has with the natural environment, traditional knowledge, and decolonized Western and non-Western science. Integrative social work is inherently transdisciplinary and recognizes that all healing and helping systems are based on evidence-guided practice. However, many integrative approaches highlight methods such as yoga, meditation, physical movement, and healthy nutrition as forms of consumerism and cultural appropriation with little or no emphasis on decolonization. This book therefore focuses on decolonizing integrative pathways to healing.

In social work literature, there has been growing recognition of the importance of alternative or complementary approaches to physical, social, and mental health (e.g., Canda, Furman, and Canda, 2019; Lee, Chan, Chan, Ng, and Leung, 2018). This emerging interest is based on many years of expanding the theoretical and practice base of social work knowledge. Already in the 1970s, the person-in-environment and ecological perspectives on social work sought to broaden biopsychosocial views by emphasizing the relationship between people and their environments (Green and McDermott, 2010). Social and community development views focused on working with neighborhoods and local institutions to enhance well-being (Taylor and Roberts, 1985). Radical and critical social work approaches challenged the power imbalances at the root of social injustice, structures of health and social welfare, and social work (Reisch and Andrews, 2001). Anti-oppressive, feminist, and ethnically sensitive practices sought to make visible how racism, sexism, and ethnocentrism often drive discriminatory policies and behaviors (Dominelli and Campling, 2014). Eco-social theories have raised questions about the anthropocentric modernist roots of social work practice, especially in relation to the environment (Boetto, 2017; Närhi, 2018). Finally, advocacy and empowerment theories promoted consciousness-raising and using power as positive resources for social change (Turner and Maschi, 2015). All of these theoretical approaches have pushed the social work conversation forward on knowledge and practices that best support the diversity of people in complex social conditions of oppression and marginalization, though decolonization has largely remained on the edges of this discourse.

The notion of integrative social work first appeared in the literature with the trailblazing *Integrative Body-Mind-Spirit Social Work: An Empirically Based Approach to Assessment and Treatment* (Lee, Chan, Chan, Ng, and Leung, 2018), a book that sought to examine how Eastern philosophies and practices could complement Western social work. There have also been explorations of the application of Daoist concepts to working with people with depression (Chan, Chan, and Chan, 2014), the use of a dialectics in multiprofessional teams (Moon, 2016), and integrative approaches to working with the survivors of family violence (Cairns-Descoteaux, 2005).

In recent decades, decolonizing social work has emerged as an attempt to broaden and critique the agenda of universalizing international social work spreading around the world (Razack, 2009). Formative texts, such as *Decolonizing Methodologies* (Smith, 2012) and *Indigenous Social Work around the World* (Gray, Coates, and Yellow Bird, 2008), have developed new vocabularies, perspectives, and approaches to address some of the most significant global trends in contemporary social work. Rooted in Indigenous worldviews and postcolonial theory (Gray, Coates, Yellow Bird, and Hetherington, 2016), decolonizing social work explores the tacit world of colonialism that is hidden in many of the assumptions, standards, and definitions of social work. These assumptions promote professional imperialism by privileging Western notions of social work over other kinds of local knowledge (Midgely, 2008; Razack, 2009). Decolonizing social work brings to the fore the significance of culturally appropriate and engaged political practice in diverse local settings (Smith, 2012). Decolonizing social work opens the door to a much more holistic understanding of the role and purpose of social work rooted in memory work and historical trauma. It includes underrepresented aspects of social work practice such as the many values of spirituality and alternative ways of healing, as well as the value of local community and family structures and practices.

Many Western countries have implemented socioeconomic policies that veer toward austerity and neoliberalism. They have removed many of the basic entitlements and social rights of citizens, shifting the role of the social worker away from its roots as an agent of social change toward one of social control by serving institutions where reimbursement shapes function (Gilbert, 1998). Though social justice remains the guiding principle of the social work profession, the often relentless focus on individualized, clinical solutions, and reliance on quantitative evidence-based data as the sole source of knowledge narrows the potential for mutuality, inclusion, and transformative change, especially in conditions (as with Fresno State) where decisions and interactions are controlled by hierarchies. The increasing relevance of Indigenous methodologies (Hertel, 2017) and decolonizing methods in the human services (Gray, Coates, and Yellow Bird, 2008) show great promise for upending settler colonial understandings of supporting vulnerable and oppressed people by fundamentally reformulating the ways that we perceive how we should do social work. These perspectives seek to empower populations long rendered invisible as experts on their own lives through Indigenous ways of healing, such as rejecting a mind–body split of knowledge, recognizing historical trauma, valuing the primacy of relationality, and cherishing memory work. Decolonizing social work thus means transforming its role as a tool of state institutions and taking it back into the community in resistance to oppressive neoliberal conditions, bearing in mind Audre Lorde's adage: "The master's tools will never dismantle the master's house."

Indigenous ways of knowing

Throughout the world, Indigenous Peoples are regarded as descended from the original nations and cultures that resided on the lands long before the advent of settler colonialism and industrial capitalism. As we discussed in our Introduction, Indigenous Peoples have occupied and settled the Americas for tens of thousands of years. In that time, the knowledge bases, perspectives, cultures, and lifestyles among these groups were incredibly diverse and complex. While some lived close to the lands in small bands of hunter-gatherers, others numbering as many as 400,000 lived in large cities such as Tenochtitlán in central Mexico. Some groups lived in forests and jungles, on the tundra, or near the sea and drew their knowledge from these environments, while others who lived on mountains, on grasslands, or in deserts created their unique practices and views of the world from these vantage points.

Indigenous ways of knowing are broad and are not centered only on what we think run counter to settler science and discoveries. In many instances, the inventions, technologies, philosophies, and innovations that many consider to be of 'Western' origin were present among Indigenous Peoples long before they were among Europeans. Though Indigeneity as a concept is inextricably linked to the history of settler colonialism and the emergence of the global extractive economy, it has its own complex histories, ontologies, and epistemologies (Kovach, 2009). It is thus important to consider Indigenous ways of knowing in their own right and not simply as a counterpoint to Western epistemologies.

In the academy, Indigenous scholars have pressed forward to disrupt the power and authority of Western intellectual traditions. Lakota scholar Vine Deloria, Jr., has often been regarded as most influential Indigenous voice in the United States since 1965 (Clark and Yetman, 2005). Shawnee/Lenape scholar Steve Newcomb wrote that Deloria, "led the way for a generation of American Indians who wanted to successfully challenge the hegemonic grip that the dominant society of the United States had over their lives, while calling into question many erroneous assumptions about Native existence" (Newcomb, 2005, A6). Yuchi member of the Muscogee Nation and a close friend and student of Deloria's, Professor Daniel R. Wildcat attributes profound influence to Deloria who "called attention to American Indian ways of knowing and knowledge not as historical artifacts, but as practical knowledge relevant to the modern world" (p. 417). Wildcat further provides his own conception of Indigeneity, writing that

> I take it as its most defining feature the sense in which the world *Indigenous* means being native to or of a place. As people around the world are forced to, enticed to, or 'freely' choose to adopt an increasingly homogenous commodity culture, what is lost are diverse local cultures situated in places, landscapes, and ecosystems they call home. Indigenization is a set of practices that results in processes in which people seriously reexamine and adopt those particular and unique cultures that emerged from the place they chose to live today. It is an acknowledgement that the old ways of living contain useful knowledge for our lives here and now.
>
> (Wildcat, 2005, 419)

The concept of Indigeneity includes a variety of peoples and cultures, but similarities in ontologies and epistemologies unite Indigeneity as a distinct framework of knowledge. Most understandings of knowledge are based upon fundamental assumptions about the world and being. For many Indigenous Peoples, subjectivity is highly contextual, relational, and place based – interconnected with the diverse elements of the universe (Kermoal and Altamirano-Jiménez, 2016). It does not maintain a difference between subject and object; rather, it approaches knowing holistically. Considering Indigeneity as a conceptual framework with distinct forms of knowledge construction raises profound questions about the nature of knowing. Viewing non-Western understandings about the nature of reality as solely cultural presumes they simply reflect variations on a singular notion of what is. Aboriginal Studies professor Mario Blaser (2014, 50) has asked: "What is knowledge in a context where the distinction between subject and object become moot?" Using settler colonial languages and conceptualizations to explore Indigeneity inevitably limits and restricts us from fully understanding the breadth and depth of Indigenous ways of knowing. As Fulvio Mazzocchi (2006, 463) points out, "Our difficulty in approaching the knowledge from indigenous cultures is already reflected in the way in which we describe and name it."

In considering Indigenous ontologies and epistemologies, we realize that we cannot return to or recapture a pure state of knowledge before extractive capitalism and settler colonialism. We also recognize that Indigenous cultures have always been dynamic, evolving, and adapting to change. The work of recognizing and restoring contemporary Indigenous ways of knowing is thus shaped by the existential trauma of settler colonialism. As we study Indigenous ways of knowing, we do so in the shadow of the experience of genocide, land theft, cultural dispossession, boarding schools, marginalization, and ongoing femicide of missing and murdered Indigenous women. We argue that reemergent Indigeneity holds the possibility to transform violent colonial forms of knowledge that seek to dominate and control. Indigenous ways of knowing offer opportunities for human liberation and a socially just futurity.

Many Indigenous Peoples around the globe have lived close and interdependent lives with the surrounding natural world. The earth, trees, animals, and ancestors coexist with the contemporaneous social formation of Indigenous societies in diverse locales. As such, Indigenous ways of knowing represent a profoundly non-anthropocentric and relational orientation to ways of being and knowing. While Western thought has commonly created a dichotomy between nature and culture, the non-human and human, Indigenous ways of thinking recognize the fundamental interplay between non-humans shaping human social life and vice versa (Kwek and Seyfert, 2018). Before industrialization and the eco-devolution of Western society, many Western tribal groups also lived close to the natural world. Now, having lost these connections, Western ways of knowing center generally on humans being located at the top of the hierarchy of existence and everything else is there to be manipulated and exploited for the benefit of humans. The paradigm of cooperation between humans and animals bears this out. Studies of domestic animals, for example, generally focus on explaining why humans decided to tame animals rather than exploring why or how animals decided to cooperate with humans (Stépanoff, 2017). This example is further detailed in the work of Andrei Golovnev and Gail Osherenko (1999), who studied the Nenets people of the Arctic, an Indigenous group that is completely interdependent with pastoral reindeer. They tell of the Nenet myth about a herd of reindeer that was attacked by wolves. The reindeer decided to join the company of people for safety and protection and thus began the path of interdependent and sustainable livelihood between the two species. In this story, the reindeer have as much agency and ability to decide as do the humans. While the myth does not 'prove' a scientific fact, it does demonstrate a fundamentally distinct ontology of mutuality and relationality in understanding behavior.

Settler colonial hierarchies often trivialize, ignore, other, or censor Indigenous ways of knowing as a 'folk practice' or 'traditional beliefs' rather than as a coherent body of knowledge. Settler ways of knowing generally center a positivist paradigm that advances the notion that ways of knowing are based on a single truth and reality. Indigenous Peoples, on the other hand, are more likely to recognize that there is no single reality. Consequently, Indigenous Peoples throughout the world have developed complex ontologies of being closely linked with place that mirror contemporary concepts of quantum physics that view the universe as constant flow that is both infinite and localized (Ferguson, 2005). While colonial societies have understood time-space and knowledge as linear, like an arrow that moves relentlessly forward, most Indigenous societies have maintained a cosmology that embraces both cyclical, natural rhythms as well as positioned, event-driven temporalities. The construction of Indigenous subjectivity is deeply interwoven with natural and spiritual environments as well as the specific circumstances of the group and its history. This mean that there is little separation between being and the elements of creation, reflecting a dynamic consciousness. The separation between subject and object is thus absurd in an Indigenous worldview, which centers relationality as a fundamental principle of all existence, which has significant implications for how being and action is understood.

Indigenous ways of knowing are embedded in complex kinship systems deeply connected to land. Knowledge has often been passed down in many Indigenous communities through oral traditions that span generations. However, these knowledge systems ways of have been challenged in a number of ways. For instance, the trauma of the reproductive injustice enacted on Indigenous women by the medical field and the removal of Indigenous children over generations by social workers and educators had a devastating impact. The erasure of cultural knowledge by assimilationist policies have placed significant barriers to traditional methods of knowledge transference in Indigenous communities. Nonetheless, examples proliferate of Indigenous resistance to the erasure of their ways of knowing. Active kinship networks of women in Aboriginal and Torres Strait Islander communities, for instance, have consciously revitalized relational and holistic ways of knowing and acting through the restoration of cultural practices that extend beyond the trauma of the colonial encounter (Dudgeon and Bray, 2019).

Indigenous knowledge has been preserved through writing systems that included the use of pictographic scripts, glyphs, paintings, and the oral tradition. In pre-Columbian Mesoamerica, as many as 15 distinct writing systems have been identified (Macri, 1996). In regard to the oral tradition, a study of the impact of human migration on fauna revealed that a close analysis of recorded Māori oral traditions stretching back to the 1500s reflected an accurate history and understanding of ecological change (Wehi, Cox, Roa, and Whaanga, 2018). This study verified for a scholarly audience that the Māori were not merely passive actors or observers of changing ecology, but the oral traditions revealed a complex interaction between cultural ideas, interactions, and practices in relation to the environment. Indigenous oral traditions have been a rich evidentiary source to understand cosmological observations (Blythe, 1992), graphic representations of history (Acuto, 2018), and ways of supporting well-being (Cumes, 2013; Koithan and Farrell, 2010). These complex oral traditions disrupt the linearity, similarity, and hierarchy of colonial ways of knowledge production.

Most important, Indigenous ways of knowing directly challenge the dominance of colonizing ways of knowing. An Indigenous framework of knowledge is intrinsically pro-Indigenous or anti-colonial because, as Ahmed Ilmi (2012, 151) points out, its ontologies and epistemologies "provide the tools to subvert and resist colonial hegemonic ideologies and discourse." For instance, Indigenous ways of knowing open up possibilities for reimagining and reconnecting the intrinsic relationality of all beings because they are not restricted by the compartmentalization of settler colonial frameworks. An Indigenous research paradigm, Shawn Wilson wrote, would recognize that "relationships don't just shape Indigenous reality, they are our reality" (2003, 173). More recently, Indigenous ontologies and epistemologies have been applied by many scholars and practitioners to critique how using Western epistemologies as the foundation of research recolonizes Indigenous communities (Said, 2019), explore how Orisha traditions in the African diaspora can support community well-being and social activism (James, 2018), and develop Indigenous standpoint theories that address the power imbalance of research and interventions driven by settler colonial-modernist scientific frameworks (Foley, 2011). The use of Indigenous ontologies and epistemologies reflects a living tradition that continues to develop and conceptualize ways of knowing, one that survived the violence of the colonial encounter.

In applying Indigenous ways of knowing to healing, we recognize that many of the Western systems developed to support health and well-being remain controlling, top-down, bureaucratic, and clinical. These settler colonial approaches tend to focus on treating individuals as diagnoses rather than communities as relational entities, and they often completely ignore the connection with environment and the cosmos. Many social welfare policies and practices continue to pathologize individuals and families who struggle with unrecognized postcolonial traumas as they are forced to assimilate into systems of care that do not recognize the connection between ill being and generational historical injustice. Different forms of knowledge construction and alternative methods and understandings of healing remain marginalized from the mainstream human services. With the growth of neoliberal evidence-based practices, settler colonial systems tend to demand submission to their own measurable processes of diagnosis and treatment, which can enhance desperation, isolation, and ill-being. When a settler colonial way of knowing is privileged over other ways of knowing, then many kinds of evidence are often overlooked and undervalued. Discussions about and practices in the human services increasingly look to narrow quantitative evidence-based models as the sole standard of validity. In this book, we use storytelling and explore diverse ways of understanding well-being to serve as a foundation for healing.

The following chapters explore how social, affective, behavioral, contemplative, and cultural elements of decolonization might be integrated into social work interventions from the community level down to the individual level, exploring how decolonizing and integrative approaches to well-being can be socially transformative.

References

Acuto, F. 2018. Understanding the Past Through Indigenous Knowledge and Archaeological Research. *Archaeologies*, 14(1): 30–61.

Blaser, M. 2014. Ontology and Indigeneity: On the Political Ontology of Heterogeneous Assemblages. *Cultural Geographies*, 21(1): 49–58.

Blythe, J. M. 1992. Climbing a Mountain Without a Ladder: Cosmology and Oral Traditions. *Time & Society*, 1(1): 13–27.

Boetto, H. 2017. A Transformative Eco-Social Model: Challenging Modernist Assumptions in Social Work. *The British Journal of Social Work*, 47(1): 48–67.

Broadhurst, K., Hall, C., Wastell, D., White, S., and Pithouse, A. 2010. Risk, Instrumentalism and the Humane Project in Social Work: Identifying the Informal Logics of Risk Management in Children's Statutory Services. *British Journal of Social Work*, 40(4): 1046–1064.

Cairns-Descoteaux, B. 2005. The Journey to Resiliency: An Integrative Framework for Treatment for Victims and Survivors of Family Violence. *Social Work and Christianity*, 32(4) (Fall): 305–320.

Canda, E. R., Furman, L. D., and Canda, H.-J. 2019. *Spiritual Diversity in Social Work Practice: The Heart of Helping*. 3rd ed. Oxford and New York: Oxford University Press.

Chan, C., Chan, T., and Chan, C. 2014. Translating Daoist Concepts into Integrative Social Work Practice: An Empowerment Program for Persons with Depressive Symptoms. *Journal of Religion and Spirituality in Social Work*, 33(1): 61–72.

Clark, D. A. T., and Yetman, N. R. 2005. "To Feel the Drumming Earth Come Upward": Indigenizing the American Studies Discipline, Field, Movement. *American Studies*, 46(3/4): 7–21.

Clayton, V. 2016. The Problem with the GRE. *The Atlantic*. Accessed 14 April 2019 at www.theatlantic.com/education/archive/2016/03/the-problem-with-the-gre/471633/

Cumes, D. 2013. South African Indigenous Healing: How It Works. *Explore: The Journal of Science and Healing*, 9(1): 58.

Dominelli, L., and Campling, J. 2014. *Anti-oppressive Social Work Theory and Practice*. Basingstoke: Palgrave Macmillan.

Dudgeon, P., and Bray, A. 2019 Indigenous Relationality: Women, Kinship and the Law. *Genealogy*, 3: 23.

Ferguson, E. 2005. *Einstein, Sacred Science, and Quantum Leaps: A Comparative Analysis of Western Science, Native Science and Quantum Physics Paradigm*. MA thesis. University of Lethbridge. Accessed at www.uleth.ca/dspace/handle/10133/253.

Foley, R. 2011. Performing Health in Place: The Holy Well as a Therapeutic Assemblage. *Health and Place*, 17(2): 470–479.

Fook, J. 2011. The Politics of Competency Debates. *Canadian Social Work Review/Revue Canadienne De Service Social*, 28(2): 295–298.

Gilbert, N. 1998. From Service to Social Control: Implications of Welfare Reform for Professional Practice in the United States. *European Journal of Social Work*, 1(1): 101–108.

Golovnev, A. V., and Osherenko, G. 1999. *Siberian Survival: The Nenets and Their Story*. Ithaca, NY: Cornell University Press.

Gray, M., Coates, J., and Hetherington, T. 2013. *Environmental Social Work*. Milton Park, Abingdon, Oxon: Routledge.

Gray, M., Coates, J., and Yellow Bird, M. (eds.). 2008. *Indigenous Social Work Around the World: Towards Culturally Relevant Education and Practice*. Aldershot: Ashgate.

Gray, M., Coates, J., Yellow Bird, M., and Hetherington, T. (eds.). 2016. *Decolonizing Social Work*. London: Routledge.

Green, D., and McDermott, F. 2010. Social Work from Inside and Between Complex Systems: Perspectives on Person-in-Environment for Today's Social Work. *British Journal of Social Work*, 40(8): 2414–2430.

Haug, E. 2005. Critical Reflections on the Emerging Discourse of International Social Work. *International Social Work*, 48(2): 126–135.

Hertel, A. L. 2017. Applying Indigenous Knowledge to Innovations in Social Work Education. *Research on Social Work Practice*, 27(2): 175–177.

Ilmi, A. 2012. Living the Indigenous Ways of Knowing: The African Self and a Holistic Way of Life. *Journal of Pan African Studies*, 4(9): 148.

James, S. 2018. Indigenous Epistemology Explored Through Yoruba Orisha Traditions in the African Diaspora. *Women & Therapy*, 41(1–2): 114–130.

Kermoal, N. J., and Altamirano-Jiménez, I. 2016. *Living on the Land: Indigenous Women's Understanding of Place*. Edmonton: Athabasca University Press.

Koithan, M., and Farrell, C. 2010. Indigenous Native American Healing Traditions. *The Journal for Nurse Practitioners*, 6(6): 477–478.

Kovach, M. 2009. *Indigenous Methodologies*. Toronto: University of Toronto.

Kwek, D., and Seyfert, R. 2018. Affect Matters: Strolling through Heterological Ecologies. *Public Culture*, 30(1): 35–59.

Lee, M. Y., Ng, S.-M., Leung, P. P. Y., and Chan, C. 2018. *Integrative Body-Mind-Spirit Social Work: An Empirically Based Approach to Assessment and Treatment*. Second edition. Oxford: Oxford University Press.

Macri, M. J. 1996. Maya and Other Mesoamerican Scripts. In *The World's Writing Systems*, edited by P. Daniels and W. Bright, 172–182. Oxford: Oxford University Press.

Margolin, L. 1997. *Under the Cover of Kindness: The Invention of Social Work*. Charlottesville: University Press of Virginia.

Mazzocchi, F. 2006. Western Science and Traditional Knowledge: Despite Their Variations, Different Forms of Knowledge Can Learn from Each Other. *Embo Reports*, 7(5): 463–466.

Midgely, J. 1981. *Professional Imperialism: Social Work in the Third World*. London: Heinemann Educational.

Midgely, J. 2008. Promoting Reciprocal International Social Work Exchanges: Professional Imperialism Revisited. In *Indigenous Social Work Around the World: Towards Culturally Relevant Education and Practice*, edited by M. Gray, J. Coates, and M. Yellow Bird, 31–45. Aldershot: Ashgate.

Moon, J. 2016. Developing Integrative Perspectives of Social Work Identity through Dialectics. *British Journal of Social Work*, 47(5) (July): 1326–1343.

Närhi, K. 2018. The Ecosocial Approach in Social Work as a Framework for Structural Social Work. *International Social Work*, 61(4): 490–502.

Newcomb, S. 2005. A Scholar's Influence in Indian Country. *Indian Country Today*, 12 January.

Payne, M., and Askeland, G. A. 2008. *Globalization and International Social Work: Postmodern Change and Challenge*. London: Ashgate.

Razack, N. 2009. Decolonizing the Pedagogy and Practice of International Social Work. *International Social Work*, 52(1) (January): 9–21.

Reisch, M., and Andrews, J. 2001. *The Road Not Taken: A History of Radical Social Work in the United States*. Philadelphia: Brunner-Routledge.

Said, S. 2019. Knowing Through Being Known: Reflections on Indigenous Epistemology and Participatory Consciousness. *Interventions*, 21(8): 1124–1138.

Smith, L. T. 2012. *Decolonizing Methodologies: Research and Indigenous Peoples*. London: Zed.

Stépanoff, C. 2017. The Rise of Reindeer Pastoralism in Northern Eurasia: Human and Animal Motivations Entangled. *Journal of the Royal Anthropological Institute*.

Taylor, S., and Roberts, R. 1985. *Theory and Practice of Community Social Work*. New York: Columbia University Press.

Turner, S., and Maschi, T. 2015. Feminist and Empowerment Theory and Social Work Practice. *Journal of Social Work Practice*, 29(2) (March): 151–162.

Wehi, P. M., Cox, M. P., Roa, T., and Whaanga, H. 2018. Human Perceptions of Megafaunal Extinction Events Revealed by Linguistic Analysis of Indigenous Oral Traditions. *Human Ecology*: 1–10.

Wildcat, D. R. 2005. Indigenizing the Future: Why We Must Think Spatially in the Twenty-first Century. *American Studies*, 46: 417–440.

Wilson, G. 2013. Evidencing Reflective Practice in Social Work Education: Theoretical Uncertainties and Practical Challenges. *British Journal of Social Work*, 43(1): 154–172.

Wilson, S. 2003. Progressing Toward an Indigenous Research Paradigm. *Canadian Journal of Native Education*, 27(2): 161–178.

4 Water

...

MICHAEL SHARES A STORY

Our planet is warming, and the ice caps are melting, causing a rise in the oceans,
which are swamping populated islands in the Pacific. More and more plastics are
ending up in the oceans, strangling sea mammals, fish, and birds, and becoming
embedded in their bodies and organs. In some parts of the world, longer and more
severe droughts are causing residents to become climate refugees as they flee their
homelands in search of new and sustainable sources of land, food, and water security. In the United States, similar to many other nations, industry, private citizens,
and governments are involved in depositing heavy metals, pesticides, pharmaceuticals, poisons, and all kinds of other contaminants into our drinking water.

Many of us in industrialized nations rarely give water a second thought. We
turn on the faucets of our showers, bathtubs, kitchen sinks, fountains, and backyard sprinklers, and without fail, water flows. When we're thirsty, we don't even
have to drink out of a public tap water source. We can stop at a market and grab
a bottle of designer water infused with all the essential vitamins and minerals and
drink to our heart's delight. We can even throw the plastic into the garbage so that
it can end up in the sea, with no penalty whatsoever.

In 2016, a major global grassroots movement began on the Standing Rock Indian
Reservation in North Dakota to stop the construction of the Energy Transfer Partner's Dakota Access Pipeline in the northern United States, which was to be built
underneath the Missouri River, the major source of drinking water for the Standing
Rock Sioux tribe and many other communities down river. The movement was
known as NoDAPL or No Dakota Access Pipeline. Fears that the pipeline could
leak and contaminate the water were deeply grounded in an eerie but highly plau-
sible reality. Refining oil sands produces an enormous amount of toxic byprod-
ucts. An expert in epidemiological healthcare research, Madelon Finkel (2018, 54)
urgently called for further research, noting the threat that may be before us:

> From an environmental perspective, there is ample evidence that pipeline
> spills and ruptures of toxic, polluting diluted bitumen has serious implica-
> tions for the surrounding land and water. From a health perspective, there is
> growing evidence to show that exposure to diluted bitumen in the short-term

causes mild to serious adverse events. The potential long-term adverse health effects are not clear, which is why comprehensive study to empirically quantify the potential harm from long-term exposure, including genotoxicity, neurotoxicity, and endocrine toxicity, is so necessary.

'Water protectors,' as they referred to themselves, rather than being regarded as protesters, engaged in nonviolent actions against the pipeline (or black serpent) peacefully marching, using Indigenous elders to perform healing ceremonies, and saying prayers for the people, the future, and the waters. On the other hand, corporate interests and the state of North Dakota (those seeking to make the pipeline a reality, with disregard for Indigenous sovereignty and cultural, human, and land rights) responded using violent and brutal tactics. State national guard units were brought in to control the highways and access into Sacred Stone Camp on the Standing Rock reservation, the site of gathering of Indigenous water protectors and their allies.

State and local police and law enforcement from other states were brought in. Private security groups that were used by the Energy Transfer Partners company operated openly and illegally in the area. The police and private security forces shot the water protectors with rubber bullets and threw concussion grenades into peaceful gatherings without regard for children, babies, and elders who were a part of the groups; from above they harassed the people using helicopters and illegally unmarked planes for surveillance and creating noise from above. Protectors were pepper sprayed, tear gassed, clubbed, beaten, and arrested; the private security company unleashed attack dogs on the elderly, women, children, and youth – exactly what police did to African Americans who were marching for civil rights, in Birmingham, Alabama, in 1963. It was horrific.

And although the civil and human rights of Indigenous Peoples and their allies were brutally violated over and over again, no one came to their aid. There was no one they could call upon for help. There was no intervention by the federal government or any group with authority that could stop the violence. It wasn't until very late in the construction of the pipeline that the Obama administration got involved to temporarily halt the construction. Indigenous Peoples and their allies also made several pleas to Hillary Clinton, the Democratic presidential candidate at that time, who was running against Donald Trump. She refused to respond and remained silent. Donald Trump, the Republican candidate for US president, was heavily invested in Energy Transfer Partners.

In the end, the efforts to protect the waters from the pipeline were not successful. Donald Trump was elected president, and he immediately signed an executive order to approve the Dakota Access Pipeline. Now Obama is gone, and so is Clinton, living their lives of privilege in relative obscurity as so many former US presidents do. Their legacies of inaction to protect the climate, the waters, and the rights of Indigenous Peoples will always be with us.

Still, there is hope. In 2018, a number of young women of color were elected to the US Congress: Ilhan Omar of Minnesota, Rashida Tlaib of Michigan, Ayanna

Pressley of Massachusetts, Sharice Davids of Kansas, Deb Haaland of New Mexico, and Alexandria Ocasio-Cortez of New York. Haaland and Davids were the first Native American women ever elected to the US Congress. Each woman has pushed for a progressive agenda including health care for all, living wages, and ideological, generational, and racial changes, demonstrating an intersectional understanding of the intrinsic connections between issues. Ocasio-Cortez, the youngest woman ever elected to Congress, was one of the main supporters of the New Green Deal, a proposal that aims to convert the present fossil fuel economy into a new, green economy that is environmentally sustainable, economically secure, and socially just. Alexandria Ocasio-Cortez joined Deb Haaland at Standing Rock. She later stated that,

> I first started considering running for Congress, actually, at Standing Rock in North Dakota. It was really from that crucible of activism where I saw people putting their lives on the line . . . for people they've never met and known. When I saw that, I knew that I had to do something more.
>
> (quoted in Solnit, 2019)

Maybe the ancestors and the waters were listening.

Remembering – 6 August 1982

For many Indigenous Peoples, water is not only life to people, animals, and plants but is also intimately tied to many other phenomena in our world and has deep spiritual meaning. In North America, many tribal peoples believe that water has an association with one or more of the four cardinal directions – north, east, south, and west. The Four Directions are important, especially with regard to understanding our place and location on Mother Earth, and there is both a practical and spiritual significance to what each direction means. In the practical sense, north is considered the direction that is up, while south is down, both in reference to the poles of the Earth. East and west are associated with Earth's rotation, that is, from east to west; the morning sun rises in the east and the evening sun sets in the west. The circadian rhythms of plants, insects, birds, animals, fish, and humans are governed by a 24-hour biological cycle based upon the rising and setting of the sun. Tides of the ocean and other bodies of water rise and fall according to the gravitational forces of the moon and sun and the rotation of the Earth.

Among the Arikara people of present-day North Dakota, the four cardinal directions (north, south, east, and west) are actually semi-cardinal directions: southeast, southwest, northwest, and northeast. Each of the directions has important spiritual significance, and each is connected to all the known forces and powers in the universe: The southeast direction represents the rising sun and all of the animal nations that walk, crawl, and move about the earth and the nations of plants, trees, flowers, and grasses, which are believed to embody similar behaviors, thoughts, and emotions as humans. The southwest is associated with all bodies of water, rain, snow, and ice, and all of the creatures that live and swim in the waters of the earth. In the northwest, we find the winds, all the celestial spirits and objects (stars and planets), and all the nations of animals that fly. Finally, the night, our dreams, and an important spiritual female deity of the Arikara, called Mother Corn, reside in the northeast direction.

On a hot summer day on a Friday afternoon following work, I was sitting outside in my backyard reflecting and journaling about my position as the human resources administrator for my tribal government. My job, as a young master of social work (MSW), was to be responsible for directly supervising several program directors and overseeing the operation of a very large social service, health, and education department. About a year and a half earlier, I had completed my MSW degree at the University of Wisconsin, Milwaukee, and had the good fortune to be in the first Native American graduate social work student cohort that was mentored by a Native American social work professor: Dr. Ronald G. Lewis (Cherokee). I learned a great deal from Dr. Lewis and, in my backyard, was reflecting on a number of things that he said to me when I was close to graduating and planning a return to my home and reservation.

I'll always remember that conversation. Dr. Lewis met me in the parking lot of the Helen Bader School of Social Welfare building to congratulate me on my completion of my degree. We talked for a long time about the courses, my peers, where some of us were headed after graduation, and of course, the future prospects for Native American people. During a brief lull in our visit, Dr. Lewis told me that since I had done exceptionally well in the program, I should stay in Milwaukee and begin work on my PhD. I was happy that he had such confidence in me, but I told him that I felt like I had had enough of the daily grind of graduate education and that I missed home and was anxious to go back so that I could see my friends, family, and relatives and to be on land and the waters that I loved. He said he understood completely since he grew up in the Cherokee Nation and often thought about his family and relatives and being home participating in cultural ceremonies.

His parting words to me were:

> Michael, you will be one of a very few American Indians with a master's of social work degree back on your reservation, and your people are going to look up to you to see how you use your education to help them out with many of the problems that show up in our communities. With everything that you have learned here, it's always important to never forget who you are, where you came from, and the knowledge of your tribal chiefs and spiritual leaders, and how your people survived and got to where they are today. Remember, they tried to wipe us out, but we're still here. There's a lot of traditional knowledge that our people have that we must use to help us out of our current predicaments. When you get home and are asked to take over or start new programs to assist your people, it's important that you remember that you can't just hang a few eagle feathers on a program and think that is an Indian program or that it's going to change things. You have to return to the stories, songs, teachings, and ceremonies of your people. These are what kept

us alive, against all odds. All these have to be part of what you are doing, otherwise it won't be any different than having mainstream social service programs that are run by outsiders.

Over the many years, Dr. Lewis' prophetic words have returned to me over and over. Now, on this hot summer afternoon, I was thinking how I might use what he had said.

I heard the sound of an approaching vehicle, looked up from my notes, and watched an old black pickup truck heading my way, kicking up dust from the gravel road as it drove towards my house. It was Grandma Grace. She was a regular evening visitor who stopped by for coffee, a snack, and a visit. I loved when she came by and shared stories about the old days. After she had parked, she walked up to where I was sitting, sat down, and asked me what I was doing. I told her that I was writing some thoughts about what I could do to make my department run better so that we could do a better job helping out our folks on the rez. I said that I was thinking about what my professor, Dr. Ron Lewis, had told me just before I came home. "What did he say?" Grandma asked. "He said that we have to rely on the wisdom of our elders in order to solve our problems and incorporate our tribal ways into the social service programs that we operate; otherwise, they are going to be just another white man program." Grandma laughed, "Geez, we have a hard enough time being Indian. How are we going to be white people? He sounds like a smart man. Is he an Indian?" she asked. "Yes, grandma. A Cherokee. The smartest Indian I ever met," I replied. She smiled and nodded her head.

I went inside and got her a snack and a pitcher of water and filled a glass so she could have a cool drink. As I walked back down the stairs to the backyard, I noticed that condensation had quickly colonized the side of the glass due to the cold temperature of the water and the heat of the late afternoon. Maybe there was a lesson here: two extremes creating something new.

Grandma was looking at the cottonwoods in the backyard as I handed her the water. She kept her gaze on the trees and said, "Look at how straight the trunks of these trees are and all the leaves on the branches. It means that they've had enough to drink and the wind has been good to them." When she finished drinking, she smiled and said, "Your water really tastes good. It tastes like spring water." I replied that my water comes from the city tap, but what she was drinking was water that I had gotten from a relative who had a spring on his property.

We sat there reminiscing about how in our different eras, when we were children, we explored different wild areas on our reservation, and found and drank from natural springs. Years later, I learned that there are a number of aquifer systems located on our traditional homelands. The source that we drank from as children is called the "White Shield aquifer," which contains very fine to coarse sand and fine to coarse gravel. Testing has classified the water in the aquifer as a sodium bicarbonate type (Cates and Macek-Rowland, 1998). Interestingly, research has shown that drinking sulphate-bicarbonate-calcium water reduces lithogenic risk (developing kidney stones), improves intestinal transit, and enables a stable body weight regardless of a high food intake (Corradini et al., 2012). Even more interesting is that many of our tribal members no longer drink from these natural sources, and the rate of kidney stones, gallstones, and obesity has risen exponentially.

I mentioned that my mom and dad often talked about how, in the past, all of the people in our tribes would collect water directly from the Missouri River and use it as their main source of drinking. Grandma Grace nodded in agreement and told some stories of how people would back their teams of horses into the water and partially submerge their wagons so they could fill up their wooden barrels with drinking water. I asked if anyone ever got sick from drinking directly from the river; she wrinkled her nose and said, "No."

Drinking 'raw water' (natural, untreated sources from mountain springs and deep ground aquifers) has become a trend in the United States. Increasingly, companies that promise to deliver raw, drinkable water are popping up. These companies maintain that that raw water has more naturally occurring essential minerals that are good for our health and bacteria that can strengthen our immune system. On the other hand, some scientists (Morris, 2008) argue that water that comes from many municipal sources is little more than treated sewage and that added chemicals such as fluoride and chlorine can increase our risk for certain kinds of cancer. Because of industrialization, urbanization, and environmental colonization, many of the natural raw water sources have been polluted and are now dangerous to directly drink from. The sources of spring and river water that Grandma Grace and I drank from were free from industrial pollution, and no doubt, because our people lived closer to the lands and drank directly from the river that contained both beneficial and possibly harmful bacteria that were not eliminated by chemicals such as chlorine, we probably had a greater diversity of gut bacteria, which according to Western science is a good thing (Mosca, Leclerc, and Hugot, 2016).

Grandma said most of the wells and springs we depend on are gone. "The river we used to drink from," she said, "is contaminated with all the farm chemicals and shit from the farm animals." When Grandma Grace was younger, there were few white settlers in our territory who were doing large-scale farming and few that were raising large domestic herds of cattle and pigs. Back when I was a youth, the farms of the settlers began to grow larger and larger on and near our tribal lands, and various chemical pesticides, herbicides, and fungicides were increasingly applied on field after field, a good deal of it ending up in our natural drinking sources.

"You know that our people believe in water spirits, Michael. There are those that live in the waters and watch over the waters. Your parents have told you those stories," Grandma Grace said. I nodded in the affirmative. "What we do to the water is what we do to ourselves and the spirits of the water that watch over it. We believe that even the animals and fish that live in the waters are related to us and have guardian spirits that watch over them. Through the spirits of the waters and the animals, we know that that water is sacred, and we must not spoil it in any way. We are taught that we should not pee, poop, or put anything in the water that is harmful; otherwise, we pay a dear price like sickness, death, and insanity."

In the Arikara creation story, as told by the Arikara spiritual leader Four Rings, all of the life in the waters is related to the people. In the beginning, the people merged from Mother Earth and began a long migration to the west. Along the way, they encountered numerous difficulties and impediments. One such obstacle was a great body of water they knew that they must cross. They proceeded onward, and some were able to successfully make it to the other side, while others were not. Those who succumbed to the waters were drowned but also became the fish and creatures of the water.

Grandma continued: "Water means a lot to us and our ancestors mention it in many of our traditional stories. Water gives life, takes life, and remakes life. Our tribes have a story of a big flood that happened to the people because we were not doing what we were supposed to do, like respecting each other and taking care of the places where we live or the animals and plants we depend on." I recalled that many cultures and religious groups have flood stories that have persisted for thousands of years. I was raised a Catholic, and so was Grandma Grace. The Catholic priest and nuns repeated many times the story of how their Christian god had exacted divine retribution upon the people by sending a flood that killed almost every human on earth, except eight people, Noah, his wife, and his three sons and their wives. Now, Grandma Grace was saying that it was not a god or deity that caused the flood, but humans themselves perished because of the disorder and chaos that they created in their own world.

We had been sitting for a long time when Grandma Grace finished speaking. She stood up and said, "Come with me; I want to show you something. Maybe it's what your Indian professor meant when he said we should not forget our ways and should include them in everything that we do." She handed me her keys, and we got into her pickup and drove down the dry, dusty road towards the river, towards the sun as it was setting in the west. We stopped and parked a short distance from the shoreline of the water and got out and walked the rest of the way. We hadn't had a lot of rain that summer, so the prairie grass was dry and crunched beneath our feet. I could smell the sage and the wet shoreline and watched a group of big white pelicans drift lazily above the water.

Grandma Grace opened the small fancy, tooled leather purse she wore on her hip and took something out and held it above the water and began to pray. When she finished, she bent forward and gently tossed it into the waters. I could see a tear in her eye. Without looking at me she said, "I prayed for the water and the spirits and the life that lives in the waters. I prayed that they would remember us when we have nothing to drink and our gardens are dry. The waters are powerful, so I prayed that they do not take any of our people. I prayed that we always remember them and that our people remember not to defile them and that we remember to feed them at the appropriate times of the seasons."

Dr. Lewis's words came back to me: returning to our teachings and ceremonies. As I looked out across the water, a tear ran from my eye.

Lessons on pathways

Mni Wiconi. Water is life.

The most striking feature of Mother Earth is the prevalence of water, which covers upwards of 70% of the planet's surface. Some scientists believe that life on

Earth first emerged from water as microorganisms and algae. Water embodies the fundamental connection between all beings on Mother Earth. Diverse Indigenous cultures throughout the world have creation stories in which the children of gods, sacred beings, and animals emerged onto land reclaimed from a watery environment. The Iroquois believed that the earth was inhabited by water animals that rescued a sky woman who fell from the clouds. The animals spread mud onto the back of a great turtle to save her. As the mud grew bigger and bigger, it became Turtle Island – the original name for North America (Mohawk and Chisholm, 1994). The Blackfeet believed water is sacred and home to divine beings (LaPier, 2017). The Qur'an states that "water is the source of all life." Christians seek spiritual rebirth through baptism in water. Water holds a central role in Shintoism, an Indigenous Japanese religion, as a symbol of purity and the origin of life. Water is symbolic of birth, emotion, harmony, continual process, and spirituality. Water deities were prevalent in ancient spirituality and often associated with fertility. Njörðr was the Nordic god of fertility, the sea, and the wind. The Taínos worshipped Atabey, the goddess of fresh water and fertility. Mermaids, mermen, and water nymphs appeared in cultures as diverse as Lithuania (Dugnė), the Philippines (Siyokoy), and the Aztec (Tlaloquetotontli). The spiritual connection between fertility, creation, sustaining life, and water as sacred emerged in many places throughout the globe simultaneously but was largely suppressed by the imposition of settler colonial institutional religions and ideologies.

Water transcends, creates, and accommodates borders or boundaries. It is in a state of constant flow and movement, falling from the sky and seeping deep into the earth before returning back into the cosmos. Water flows by gravity and topography and rarely follows a straight line. The streamflow of rivers is always changing depending on water levels and gravity. Land acts as a watershed distributing rainwater and snowmelt to groundwaters, soil, and rivers, which journey to the ocean. Seeping water will eventually soften and reshape even the hardest of elements, such as stone or cement. Fast-moving, large torrents of water can flood and when combined with wind can reshape the landscape and overwhelm the living things in its path. Flooding can have a profound impact on the environment in both positive and negative ways. It can redistribute organic materials, trigger bird breeding events, and cause deep sedimentation in marine systems. There are often devastating social consequences to humans from flooding. In 1931, Huang He (also known as the Yellow River) flooded, killing as many as four million people. Huang He is thus often referred to as 'China's Sorrow' because of the high death tolls its flooding has caused. Conversely, the Egyptians had a very different relationship with the Nile River: When flooding occurred, they referred to it as the 'Gift of the Nile,' since the waters spread a very fertile, rich black mud that was critical for planting a successful and abundant crop.

The vast majority of the Earth's surface is water in the form of rivers, lakes, oceans, and glaciers. Water is an essential element of homo sapiens. At birth, humans are 90% water, which is eventually reduced to 70% in middle age. The brain and the heart are made up of 73% water, and even our bones consist of 31% water. We can go without food for weeks, but we must consume water every three days to survive. Water is the fundamental life force without which we shrivel and die.

Settlers used water as a means to travel to new lands to explore, settle, and colonize. Colonialism brought a fundamentally altered relationship to the sense of place and water. Water is perhaps the most significant factor in human settlement. As settlers invaded Indigenous territories, they set about manipulating and controlling the waterways for their own benefit: They began damming up rivers and streams to create a permanent source of water; they settled near and controlled prime locations near waterways, keeping out Indigenous Peoples and displacing the natural flora and fauna that depended on the water; to build their farms, towns, and cities; and they diverted water from streams and rivers. To colonize, remake, and take control of the territories they invaded, settlers began using major waterways as their routes of commerce, transporting goods from town to town and to coastal locations.

Settler use of Indigenous waterways proved exceptionally deadly for Indigenous Peoples. The Great Plains smallpox epidemic of 1837 that killed as many as 17,000 Indigenous Peoples (Daschuk, 2013) came by way of a steamboat named the *St. Peter* traveling up the Missouri River. One of the deckhands was infected with the disease as were some of the blankets on the boat. Indigenous Peoples had no immunity to many European diseases, and smallpox proved to be the deadliest. The Mandan were the hardest hit. In the spring of 1837, there were about 2,000 Mandan people living in the Knife River villages along the Missouri River. By October, only 138 remained alive.

During the early days of the Industrial Revolution, many died of waterborne illnesses due to poor sanitation. It was common for residents to throw refuse, wash clothes, and discard dead animals in water sources such as the Thames and Seine Rivers. Throughout the early nineteenth century, there were waves of cholera outbreaks that took thousands of lives in London and parts of New York City. Industrial cities were filthy with overcrowded tenements and no indoor plumbing. Early social work informed the herculean efforts of public health, civil engineering, housing, and public officials to design community water systems that ensured the safe disposal of waste and access to clean water essential to support vast industrial cities. By the mid-twentieth century, waterborne illnesses were rare. For nearly a century, people in the industrialized world have been accustomed to safe and plentiful water flowing through taps. We use water for our lawns, car washes, infant formula, to refine gasoline, to grow food, and to make plastic water bottles. Nowadays, if a North American family does not have clean running water, then children can be subject to removal by child welfare workers on the basis of neglect. Water is therefore at the heart of social work.

In her ethnography of addiction and dispossession in New Mexico, Angela Garcia writes that there is a high cost to the commodification and privatization of this vital resource (Garcia, 2010). In the case that Garcia relates, the displacement of Indigenous People from their traditionally integrative and communal relationship to water and land in the mid-twentieth century resulted in disrupted communities, unemployment, and ultimately despair and addiction by the turn of the millennium. The overarching issue of the significance of water, land, and community was lost in social work interventions by focusing solely on the minutiae of managing drug use among Indigenous Peoples rather than seeing that drug use was only a symptom of the loss of water, land, and community. Missing the bigger picture of the structural web of causality meant that treating symptoms and side effects would inevitably lead to failed stints at rehabilitation. When the Péligre Dam was constructed in Haiti, it led to the widespread displacement as people's rural livelihoods were destroyed and they were forced to migrate to the cities. Beyond the social disruption, significant negative health outcomes resulted from the entire process surrounding the dam project, increasing tuberculosis and HIV rates in particular (Farmer, 2006). As water has become a commodity to control, the fundamentally integrative relationship of people with their environment has been broken, causing harm to both people and water.

In the twenty-first century, there are increasing barriers to clean and plentiful water due to neoliberal ideologies, austerity measures, the privatization of water companies, and the pollution of groundwater through fracking, pesticides, and other operations. Droughts and floods are becoming ever more common with climate change. Agricultural pumps dig ever deeper into diminishing aquifers. The Navaho Nation, for example, has been plagued by a multitude of environmental and health issues due to the contamination of water by uranium drilling between 1944 and 1986. Recent coal mining has further degraded the water supply, leaving up to 30% of Navaho people with no access to regulated drinking water (Lynette, 2010). Aging industrial infrastructures and poorly maintained water systems have caused an increase in pathogens and waterborne illnesses (Morris, 2008). Harmful algal blooms, which produce toxins that can cause severe illness in humans, animals, and the local ecology, have become increasingly common globally due to climate crisis. All of these issues are making water an ever more precious resource as the centuries-long barrage of pollutants, diversion projects, and overuse systematically undermines the viability of lakes, rivers, and oceans (Morris and Spivak, 2010).

The link between lack of access to clean water and ill-being can be seen across the world. African women have traditionally been the guardians of water across the continent. With growing water scarcity, many African women must spend a disproportionate amount of time hauling heavy containers of water for ever longer distances. Even in Ireland, a nation famous for its rain, people face water charges because the government's European creditors demanded that Irish residents must start paying for water, which most Irish consider a sacred human right. The San Joaquin Valley of California is a region that produces a huge proportion of American food by way of colonial labor system that has drastically manipulated a desert environment into a growing region of monocultural agriculture. The farmworkers in this carefully controlled arrangement struggle with health issues due to long working hours and exposure to agricultural chemicals and live in areas with virtually no access to clean water. These diverse yet similar global circumstances exemplify conditions of structural violence in which institutions and structures deny people safe access to the most basic of human needs (Farmer, 2003). Economist Amartya Sen (1999) calls this structural violence "unfreedom," meaning that when basic needs are not met, then civil and political freedoms cannot be achieved. The commodification of water fractures our primal connection to the source of all life, sparking a chain reaction that results in unequal access and pollution.

Water is a basic social work issue because human beings cannot exist without it. Social work interventions in the future will be more deeply involved with disasters and population dislocation caused by the lack of water due to climate crisis. The field of social work should address the issue of water through increased advocacy for access to clean water and policies that support a non-anthropocentric respect and care for Mother Earth. We do not call for social work stewardship of our aquatic ecosystems because notions of stewardship are deeply entrenched in colonial management (Funari and Mourad, 2016); rather, we call for a deep alliance with Indigeneity and Traditional Ecological Knowledge (Popova, 2014; Ruiz-Mallén and Corbera, 2013; Zapf, 2005).

Decolonization begins when communities stand up and reject the structures imposed by settler colonial ideologies. Communities are organizing to preserve their basic human rights to clean water and the intrinsic right of water to exist without being manipulated and polluted. Following the wisdom of the ancestors, as Michael's story points out, is becoming a life or death decision. We can see this from places as far flung as Standing Rock, North Dakota, to Dublin, Ireland, to India to Flint, Michigan, to rural Kenya. The complex and calamitous threats to clean water range from oil drilling to austerity measures to contamination through pollutants to the pumping of groundwater for privatized bottled water. As social workers, we must turn our attention to what this basic element means, which is so fundamental to our existence, and how it has been put in jeopardy. We must find ways to work with individuals and communities to decolonize the exploitation of vital resource and regain our sacred relationship with water. We must recognize the fundamental right of water to exist without pollutants, diversion, and commodification. And we must explore holistic ways to integrate water into our practice. This chapter proceeds by considering how to decolonize water through an Indigenous approach and then explores the power of water to heal through the example of holy wells in Ireland.

Decolonizing our relationship of dominance over water

To decolonize our relationship of dominance over water in social work, we must begin with the recognition of historically rooted Indigenous knowledge, leadership, and action on contemporary water issues. Transforming how we understand the scope and meaning of social work theory and action thus must be co-created in dialogue with Indigenous perspectives and voices.

Indigenous cultures embody a shared and sustainable relationship to place and all of creation associated with it, including animals, water, lands, plants, spirits, and all-natural phenomena. As we discussed in Chapter 3, Indigenous ontology is enmeshed in relationality with Mother Earth subverting the Western subject–object dichotomy through its focus on the inherent significance of relationships (Kermoal and Altamirano-Jimenez, 2016). Though often misrepresented as fixed and unchanging or as simple folk knowledge, Indigenous systems of knowledge provide nimble and nuanced understandings of evolving environments as many scientists are beginning to recognize. Blackfoot elder Narcisse Blood spoke of places as being spiritual and alive and acting as our teachers (Kovach, 2009, 61). Indigenous knowledges are unique and local, making little distinction between the intrinsic value of rocks, water, human beings, fauna, and animals because all of creation is alive and interconnected. Water in an Indigenous paradigm exists as a flow from evaporation to rain to groundwater as a life cycle that must be nurtured. As Anishinaabe nation member Deborah McGregor (2008, 27) notes:

> In attempting to express the meaning of water as a discrete concept, we risk obscuring the meaning that is associated with water in traditional Aboriginal philosophies. For many Aboriginal people and their ways of life, water offers 'life giving' forces, accompanied by certain duties and responsibilities (none of which can be adequately expressed in a report). This knowledge must be lived to have meaning.

Indigenous ways of knowing thus regard water as a primal and life-sustaining force requiring vigilance, responsibility, and careful tending and not solely as a commodity to be used. Exploring different dimensions of the relationship between humans and the basic elements of Mother Earth is key to integrative social work. As noted in the first chapter's historical grounding of modern social work, the rise of the persecuting society in Europe brought a settler colonial paradigm that shifted knowing and healing from a collective approach to institutional forms of disciplinary practices. Natural elements, such as water, were no longer viewed as alive and part of the relationality of humans to their environment and were pushed outside of the purview of the social professions. As Metzner (2017, 107) notes, the Western view was limited to "the material world [that is] inert, insentient, and nonspiritual, [where] no kind of psychic or spiritual communion between humans and Earth or nature is possible."

Indigenous Peoples have always felt a responsibility to sustain water and have led resistance to colonizing efforts to privatize and commodify water resources from the first incursions on their lands by settlers. In New Zealand, Māori people have struggled to assert their water rights in the face of strong opposition from the petrochemical and fishing industries. In Finland, Skolt Sámi people have struggled to maintain traditional management practices of the salmon of the Näätämö River against the polluting impact of hydroelectric plants. Anishinaabe women have led a Mother Earth Water Walk in which people walk over 500 miles around Lakes Ontario and Erie to raise awareness about the importance of water. Started by Elder Josephine Mandamin in 2003, Anishinaabe women have used Indigenous ceremonies to unite diverse people to commit themselves for three months to protect water. Women carry copper vessels filled with water from place to place during the walk to represent the importance of protecting water. In recognizing the intrinsic rights to sustainable clean and healthy water, Indigenous Peoples are asserting water's right to exist as natural and clean by raising awareness about the toll of colonization on ourselves but also on nature, which also has a fundamental right to exist.

Decolonizing our relationship with water begins with reimagining social work theory, which continues to be constructed along anthropocentric settler colonial binaries, to be more inclusive of sacred landscapes and elements. The belief in settler dominion over nature has deep roots in the colonial experience of removing Indigenous Peoples from lands and waters that they felt were not being appropriately 'used.' We must ask ourselves if our colonized attitudes towards water are what is desirable when we use water as a dumping site for our garbage, plastics, pesticides, pharmaceuticals, and chemicals. To get past this mindset, the interrogation of social work education is essential. The current paradigm inculcates students with the notion that humans are the center of the universe and that the natural world is there to be manipulated and consumed. The human behavior in the social environment concept, for example, focuses on the individual behaviors of people in various social contexts but largely disregards the significant role of nature in our lives. Our view and use of water as a mere, convenient resource is colonized, aberrant thinking. To decolonize our relationship, it is important to recognize that water has sentience. It knows what is it doing; it knows how to respond to changes; and it will take care of us, if we take care of it.

For now, we live generally unconcerned and comfortable in the eye of the storm of climate crisis. But the calm will not last, and for those of us who came into this discipline to be agents of change, this reality is very troubling and unfortunate, for only now has social work theory begun to consider how people are rooted in contexts deeper than the social environment. Decolonizing approaches should make clear to us that there are no great social work movements today that are socially, politically, or culturally engineering us towards practice interventions and policies to stem the assault on our Mother Earth. Only now, as the climate crisis increasingly has an impact on peoples' everyday lives, some researchers have begun to examine and advocate for social work policy and practice shifts that more broadly address the worlds beyond the social environment in which we live. This is important since social work scholars like Rebecca Molyneaux (2011, 62) have observed that, "Overwhelmingly, the literature acknowledged the historically shallow relationship endorsed by the social work profession between humans and the natural realm."

Recognition of the broader dimensions and interconnections of human and natural life is key to opening up holistic pathways between social work and active resistance to contemporary settler colonialism on the structural, community, and individual levels. Beyond changing our frameworks of knowledge and understanding, decolonizing water requires reimagining practical action by social workers to deeply engage with community activism on their own terms. The complex issues surrounding water – from the lack of access to clean and affordable drinking water to climate-change impacts such as drought and hurricanes to reforming water laws to embracing the healing properties of water – all fall within the realm of social work practice. While we as social workers focus on treating the symptoms and outcomes of water issues, such as lead poisoning or displacement due to flooding, we are far too often absent at the source of the problem, namely, respect for water than commodifying it. Social work should be present at policy discussions on water management, preparations for climate crisis, and standing in solidarity with those resisting the denigration of our water. We can also restore healing practices associated with water. Embodying true cultural humility means that social work could learn from the leadership and activism of Indigenous Peoples on water issues.

Social work as a field has been increasingly engaged with issues surrounding climate crisis and water, particularly in connection with environmental injustice, as evidenced by the Grand Challenges for Social Work Initiative by the American Academy of Social Work (Kemp and Palinkas, 2015). Social workers around the globe have also launched grassroots initiatives. Agoramoorthy and Hsu (2015) writes of a social work project in India that focused on enhancing small farmers' access to irrigation water by developing participatory projects that developed community collectives to direct water projects. Robert Case (2017) discusses water activism in Canada as an example of how social workers should be engaged with building community resilience. A Cuban research project argued for the need to see water as a social resource (Hernández and Domínguez, 2014). Integrating these types of community initiatives into social work practice with a non-anthropocentric approach is key to decolonizing our relationship with water.

The government of New Zealand recently recognized the legal personhood and fundamental rights of the Whanganui River, the country's third longest river. Having nearly killed the river through pollution, New Zealanders are beginning to listen to the Indigenous Māori, who have always believed in the sacredness of water and need to preserve this vital resource for future generations. This legal precedent reflects an act of recognition of the primal significance of water in our lives as a source of life and societal well-being. Social work needs to stand with Indigenous People at the forefront of efforts to shift the colonial paradigm of how we think about and interact with our aquatic ecosystems in terms of policy and practice.

Water and healing

In the opening stories, we saw how Indigenous knowledge and relationality with water have been ignored and even lost to our great peril, as Grandma Grace sadly observed. Our water has become polluted and contaminated. Dr. Lewis's prophetic words to Michael, cautioning him to remember the wisdom of his people, was put into practice through the protests at Standing Rock. Water defenders approached threat of toxic pollution in their aquifer from an integrative and decolonizing perspective building community resilience. In linking the sacred with the everyday and utilitarian, water defenders recognized how treating this valuable resource as a commodity is destroying our communities. They further acknowledge the obligation of humans to defend water against the onslaught of extractive capitalism to preserve our common heritage. Communal holy wells weave a healing connection between ancient Indigenous culture and contemporary life through a therapeutic landscape.

Many languages have a variety of terms to describe distinct bodies of water. In the English language alone, we have many words, including spring, tributary, loch, gulf, cove, lake, pond, and bayou, among others. The extraordinary detail that we have developed through human language to describe the complexity of bodies of water reflects its significance in our everyday lives. Indeed, the annihilation of our rich vocabulary of English words about nature reflects our diminishing connection with our environment.

Water has traditionally been used to soak in, relax next to, and imbibe. It is a vital element that produces calm and wonder and heals. Water veneration (or hydrolatry) was prevalent throughout the ancient world as we pointed out earlier. In his book, *The Blue Mind*, (2015) Wallace Nichols draws on evidence to show that being near water creates a 'blue mind' at ease and increases our physical, social, and psychological well-being. He argues that just as medical practitioners are beginning to recognize the importance of integrative practices such as exercise, diet, and stress reduction techniques, being near or in water will also be viewed as holistic pathway to healing. Wallace Nichols defines 'blue mind' as a mildly meditative state characterized by tranquility and happiness (Nichols, 2015, 6).

Water creates what is called a 'therapeutic landscape' in the literature, meaning that proximity or exposure to water can lead to an embodied sense of well-being (Bell, Phoenix, Lovell, and Wheeler, 2015). According to Gesler (1996, 96), a therapeutic landscape "arises when physical and built environments, social conditions and human perceptions combine to produce an atmosphere which is conducive to healing. The term healing is used here in a broad manner to include cures in the biomedical sense (physical healing), a sense of psychological well-being (mental healing) and feelings of spiritual renewal (spiritual healing)." There are four components that make a therapeutic landscape a healing place: the natural, the built, the symbolic, and the social (Gesler, 2003). Conradson (2005) further clarifies that therapeutic landscapes are not simply the essential qualities of a place but embody relational qualities between the beholder and the space. These relational qualities are linked by cultural narratives and social meanings, such as penance or pilgrimage, and are generally assigned to a physical place.

Water and place are commonly enmeshed in culture and strongly intertwined in a therapeutic landscape, particularly when tied with ways of grappling with penance or grief (Gesler, 1996). In *Holy Ground, Healing Water: Cultural Landscapes at Waconda Lake, Kansas* (2010), Donald Blakeslee discusses the shifting geography of a sacred Indigenous spring. Waconda spring was once an ancient place where Indigenous Peoples came to communicate with the animal spirits in the spiritual world and which was handed off from one tribe to the next with its spiritual legacy intact. When settlers came to the area, they commodified the lands, altered the space, and destroyed the spiritual sacredness and legacy. Indigenous Peoples were driven out, and the bison were hunted to extinction. By 1870, Waconda spring had been stripped of its cultural meaning and turned into a resource where salt was extracted. Later, it became a sanatorium and spa for the wealthy and was ultimately bulldozed and closed up. The fate of Waconda spring is emblematic of a settler colonial approach to our most precious resource: find and expel the residents, alter the space and import invasive values and ideas, hoard and privatize the environment, exploit and destroy, repeat.

How can we preserve water as healing for all and not just a commodified place for the wealthy few? A healing space common throughout Ireland provides a model.

In Ireland, holy wells have deep roots in the ancient world of the Celts and Indigenous People of the island. Holy wells are springs or other small bodies of water that have been believed to have healing qualities for thousands of years. Holy wells are most commonly marked with a pile of stones, a cairn, and a thorn trees, which are thought to have medicinal and supernatural properties. According to the eleventh-century *Lebor Gabála Érenn* (*The Book of Invasions*), a text often viewed more as national epic than factual history, the native people of Ireland were forced underground by the invading and mythical race of Milesians, causing the Indigenous Irish people to become subterranean fairies. Thorn trees are also known as 'fairy trees' because it is believed that that's where the fairies live and meet. Contemporary roads have even been diverted to protect thorn trees as uprooting them is considered to cause bad luck. Visitors often leave bits of cloth or personal items tied to the branches, which are then termed 'rag trees.' This practice is similar to Tibetan Buddhists and Native Americans, who both hang colorful cloth prayer flags in trees and bushes to symbolize blessing, good will, compassion, and sacredness. These scraps of clothing of the Irish represent a wish or aspiration for healing or well-being. Rosaries, saints' medal or cards, and crosses also adorn the sites of holy wells.

It is estimated that there are up to 3,000 holy wells spread across Ireland (Carroll, 1999). Ray (2011) argues that there is evidence of pre-Christian water veneration, while Carroll (1999) asserts that holy wells were a post-Reformation assertion of Irish Catholicism and an important marker of identity that served a signifying purpose during the time of colonization by the British. Ray sees holy wells as part of the sacred landscape of pre-Christian Ireland and points to the high prevalence of pre-Christian origins of holy sites like the rest of Europe. As a traditional site of pilgrimage, people would perform rounding rituals, which involved walking in circles around the well. In pre-Christian times, these circles followed the journey of the sun; later they came to reflect the stations of the cross. Irish pilgrimage differed from European focus on saints with in its focus on the locus between geography and place (Cassidy, 2017). During colonization, visits to holy wells were forbidden by the British in an effort to eradicate Catholic worship, though this policy was virtually impossible to enforce. As Cassidy notes (2017, 18): "People reverted to following a landscape-based folk tradition that had never completely died out. This tradition was based on two forms: pilgrimage to difficult to access sites such as Croagh Patrick and Lough Derg, and 'patterns held at local holy wells.'" Ancient Celts found the spiritual in landscapes – mountaintops, caves, and springs – a connection which deepened Irish resistance to the British rule.

Anthropological, archaeological, and sociological perspectives on holy wells (Foley, 2011; Ray, 2011; Walsham, 2012) have in part focused on the complexity of symbols and rituals for healing through history. Ronan Foley (2010) writes of holy wells as a 'therapeutic landscape' which reflect cultural and place meanings associated with water falling into contemporary literature on therapeutic landscapes, such as community gardens and natural habitats. Holy wells continue to be popular places in Ireland for reflection and contemplation. The Republic of Ireland is a modern multicultural country that reveres most of the same Western values as its fellow European countries, such as individualism and autonomy, even as it has emerged from a complex history of Indigenous cultures, invasions, and settler colonialism. The brassy materialism of the economic boom in Ireland coexists with new immigrants, the working poor, and New Age visitors seeking Celtic alchemy in tourist spots.

About a mile from Kildare Town down the Tully Road is the St. Brigid's holy well. There is a small sign that indicates the way down a narrow lane. Like many other holy wells, the Kildare example is firmly rooted in the local – in this case, the Indigenous Brigid, a pre-Christian goddess. Later considered a patron saint of the Irish people along with St. Patrick, Brigid has traditionally been associated with fire and light. The remains of Brigid's fifth-century fire pit can be found in the grounds of a local Church of Ireland cathedral, which was built on the site of her monastery. The monastery continued to tend Brigid's fire until its suppression in the sixteenth century. The town of Kildare grew up around the monastery and later grew as the British established a military base nearby. As both a pre-Christian figure and Catholic saint, Brigid came to represent nature, fire, motherhood, purity, culture, wisdom, fertility, and healing. The Kildare holy well is bounded by a small stream and has a statue of Brigid, a small platform for donations and candles, a little footbridge across the water, and several rag trees. Rag trees are often found near holy wells and people hang scraps of clothing as tokens of their hopes on branches. It is believed that as the rag rots, the aspiration will come to fruition. Any visit to the Kildare holy well makes evident that it continues to serve as a quiet spot for contemplation. Despite their many historical iterations and complex and discontinuous cultural narratives, holy wells in Ireland continue to use water as a communal therapeutic landscape for healing.

References

Agoramoorthy, G., and Hsu, M. 2015. Irrigation-based Social Work Relieves Poverty in India's Drylands. *International Social Work*, 58(1): 23–31.

Bell, S. L., Phoenix, C., Lovell, R., and Wheeler, B. W. 2015. Seeking Everyday Wellbeing: The Coast as a Therapeutic Landscape. *Social Science & Medicine*, 142(C): 56–67.

Carroll, M. P. 1999. *Irish Pilgrimage, Holy Wells and Popular Catholic Devotion*. Baltimore: The Johns Hopkins University Press.

Case, R. A. 2017. Environmental Oversight and the Citizen Activist: Lessons from an Oral History of Activism Surrounding Elmira, Ontario's 1989 Water Crisis. *Community Development*, 48(1): 86–104.

Cassidy, J. 2017. *The Pilgrimage of Dabhach Phádraig: Place, Memory, and Sacred Landscape at the Holy Well of Belcoo*. Master's thesis. Liberal Arts. Empire State College, State University of New York.

Cates, S. W., and Macek-Roland, K. M. 1998. *Water Resources of the Fort Berthold Indian Reservation, West-Central North Dakota*. US Department of the Interior, US Geological Survey. U.S Department of The Interior. Accessed 10 November 2019 at https://pubs. usgs.gov/wri/1998/4098/report.pdf.

Conradson, D. 2005. Landscape, Care and the Relational Self: Therapeutic Encounters in Rural England. *Health and Place*, 11(4): 337–348.

Corradini, S. G., Ferri, F., Mordenti, M., Sicilliano, M., Burza, M. A., Sordi, B., Caciotti, B., Pacini, M., Santis, A. D., Roda, A., Colliva, C., and Attili, A. F. 2012. Beneficial Effect of

Sulphate-bicarbonate-calcium Water on Gallstone Risk and Weight Control. *World Journal of Gastroenterology*, 18(9) (March): 930–937.

Daschuk, J. 2013. *Clearing the Plains: Disease, Politics of Starvation, and Loss of Aboriginal Life*. Regina: University of Regina Press.

Farmer, P. 2003. *The Uses of Haiti*. Monroe, ME: Common Courage Press.

Farmer, P. 2006. *AIDS and Accusation: Haiti and the Geography of Blame*. Berkeley: University of California Press.

Finkel, M. L. 2018. The Impact of Oil Sands On the Environment and Health. *Current Opinion in Environmental Science & Health*, 3: 52–55.

Foley, R. 2010. Performing Health in Place: The Holy Well as a Therapeutic Assemblage. *Health and Place*, 17(2): 470–479.

Funari, P. P. A., and Mourad, T. O. 2016. Stewards of Empire: Heritage as Colonialist Booty. *Heródoto*, 1(1).

Garcia, A. 2010. *The Pastoral Clinic: Addiction and Dispossession Along the Rio Grande*. Berkeley: University of California Press.

Gesler, W. 1996. Lourdes: Healing in a Place of Pilgrimage. *Health and Place*, 2(2): 95–105.

Gesler, W. 2003. *Healing Places*. Oxford: Rowman and Littlefield.

Hernández, R. V., and Domínguez, D. L. 2014. Think of Water from a Social Perspective. A Research Project in Havana. *Procedia – Social and Behavioral Sciences*, 132(C): 473–478.

Kemp, S. P., and Palinkas, L. A. (with Wong, M., Wagner, K., Reyes Mason, L., Chi, I., . . . Rechkemmer, A.). 2015. *Strengthening the Social Response to the Human Impacts of Environmental Change (Grand Challenges for Social Work Initiative Working Paper No. 5)*. Cleveland, OH: American Academy of Social Work and Social Welfare.

Kermoal, N. J., and Altamirano-Jiménez, I. 2016. *Living on the Land: Indigenous Women's Understanding of Place*. Edmonton: Athabasca University Press.

Kovach, M. 2009. *Indigenous Methodologies*. Toronto: University of Toronto.

LaPier, R. 2017. *Why Is Water Sacred to Native Americans?* Open Rivers: Rethinking Water, Place & Community. No. 8.

Lynette, J. 2010. Navajo Nation: 30% Without Access to Regulated Drinking Water. *American Water Works Association Journal*, 102(10): 28–29.

McGregor, D. 2008. Anishinaabe-Kwe, Traditional Knowledge, and Water Protection. *Canadian Woman Studies*, 26(3/4): 26–30.

Metzner, R. 2017. *Ecology of Consciousness: The Alchemy of Personal, Collective, and Planetary Transformation*. Oakland, CA: New Harbinger Publications, Inc.

Mohawk, J., and Chisolm, L. W. 1994. *A View from Turtle Island: Chapters in Iroquois Mythology, History and Culture*. ProQuest Dissertations and Theses.

Molyneux, R. 2011. The Practical Realities of Ecosocial Work: A Review of the Literature. *Critical Social Work*, 11(2): 61–69.

Morris, R. 2008. *The Blue Death: The Intriguing Past and Present Danger of the Water You Drink*. New York: Harper Collins.

Morris, R. C., and Spivak, G. C. 2010. *Can the Subaltern Speak?: Reflections on the History of an Idea*. New York: Columbia University Press.

Mosca, A., Leclerc, M., and Hugot, J. P. 2016. Gut Microbiota Diversity and Human Diseases: Should We Reintroduce Key Predators in Our Ecosystem? *Frontiers in Microbiology*, 7: 455.

Nichols, W. J. 2015. *The Blue Mind*. New York: Little Brown.

Popova, U. 2014. Conservation, Traditional Knowledge, and Indigenous Peoples. *American Behavioral Scientist*, 58(1): 197–214.

Ray, C. 2011. The Sacred and the Body Politic at Ireland's Holy Wells. *International Social Science Journal*, 62(205–206): 271–285.

Ruiz-Mallén, I., and Corbera, E. 2013. Community-Based Conservation and Traditional Ecological Knowledge: Implications for Social-Ecological Resilience. *Ecology and Society*, 18(4): 12.

Sen, A. 1999. *Development as Freedom*. New York: Knopf.

Solnit, R. 2019. Standing Rock Inspired Ocasio-Cortez to Run. That's the Power of Protest. *The Guardian*, 14 January.

Walsham, A. 2012. *The Reformation of the Landscape: Religion, Identity, and Memory in Early Modern Britain and Ireland*. Oxford: Oxford University Press.

Zapf, M. K. 2005. The Spiritual Dimension of Person and Environment: Perspectives From Social Work and Traditional Knowledge. *International Social Work*, 48(5): 633–642.

5 Creative expression

Creative expression is an ancient affective language of humans, animals, and many other forms of life. From paleolithic cave art to petroglyphs to contemporary art, human beings have used the arts for millennia to express visions, spirituality, love, hope, and despair. Creative expression is the process of engaging with innovative, unconscious, and fresh thoughts and emotions, experimenting with sound, and reconnecting with the ancient while thinking and exploring feelings through tactile methods of fabricating and making. Though there are debates about the role of intentionality and value in the process and outcome of creation, creativity can be viewed as bringing into existence new or novel ideas, things, or artifacts (Harrington, 2018). Art, music, and other forms of creative expression speak to collective as well as personal aspirations, experiences, and meanings. Music's combination of vibrating sounds can evoke profound experiences in the listener. Similarly, visual art is a primal element of individual expression and cultural identity.

Research indicates that humans have a fundamental need to create for social recognition and to communicate (Zaidel, 2014). People engaged in a creative act often attain a state of 'flow' in which they have total focus, a merging of action and awareness, an altered sense of time, a lack of self-consciousness, and an intrinsic sense of reward (Cseh, Phillips and Pearson, 2015). Art and music have supported people in the most abject circumstances to survive and find meaning. The evolution of African American music from slave songs to blues to jazz to hip hop, for example, has been a way of understanding life, interweaving cultural identity with historical resilience through art (Beşe, 2012). Creative expression details our ancestral paths and historical trauma but also gives wings to the beauty and wonder of our existence and futurity.

Art and music are universal languages, but they may have specifically local dialects. The sense and meaning of visual representation can vary widely among cultures, groups, and historical periods. There are also distinct cultural forms of musicality that are connected with the way that we learn our physical and emotional cues towards music. Lullabies in Finland and Iran, for example, are often in the minor tone, which many people in other Western countries may interpret emotionally as sad compared with the major tone prevalent in their children's songs. These different orientations towards music from infancy result in distinct cultural and emotional relationships to music and expressions of musicality. The field of musical cognition, for example, explores how enculturation has an impact on the diverse emotional and cognitive responses to music. Some studies suggest that infants under one year of age have already been enculturated into specific musical meters and tones (Stalinski and Schellenberg, 2012). Our sense of creative expression is shaped with and through our kin and ancestors as well as culture and environment. The point where the physical and relational dimensions of expression coalesce at making sense of art and music has been called "embodied enculturation" (Thyssen and Grosnevor, 2019). Complicated entanglements of history and culture and the sensory experience of expression go beyond the intellectual and are relational and emotional, touching our souls.

Creative expression encapsulates many of the healing themes that we discuss here. Like the other elements in this book, creative expression is a means to help us grow and develop through our own individual relationality with others in the act of communicating imaginative ideas through material, visual, or aural form. This chapter is constructed around three different stories. The first illustrates how music is used for the colonial war machine, the second looks at how schooling is interwoven with artistic representations to reinforce colonialism, and finally the last story shows how creative expression can support resilience over generations.

Music as war machine

Kris shares a story

The rhythm and pitch of music are uniquely evocative, affecting our emotions and even movement. Indeed, music has been interwoven with colonial military identity and action through marches, cadences, parades, and ceremonies stretching back to the Roman Empire. In 2014, the US Department of Defense was the largest employer of musicians in the country with over 6,000 musicians in active duty, reserve, and the National Guard (Gleason, 2015). The quickstep marching song *Garryowen* is often played at gatherings in the United States to great acclaim and handclapping. Many find it to be an infectious tune with a cheerful beat and associate it with merry Irishmen and benign flag waving. It is hard not to tap your toes when the snare drums rattle and the flutes trill. *Garryowen* has been a staple at military parades and with marching bands in the United States for many decades.

Garryowen is an old Irish drinking song. It is thought that the tune originated as a marching song by the Royal Irish Regiment that fought for King William of Orange and was based in Limerick, Ireland, where Garryowen is a suburb. Sung by wealthy young men who ran riot and drank, the song was quickly adopted by various colonial military regiments. It was brought to settler colonial America by Irish immigrants, and the tune became an official regimental marching song starting in New York with the Irish Volunteers and was later adopted by Custer's Seventh Cavalry.

As settler colonialism pushed westward through the 'Indian Wars' of the nineteenth century, the Seventh Cavalry expanded the grip of settler colonialism by attacking Sioux and Cheyenne villages with the aim of neutralizing Indigenous resistance. When gold was discovered, settler colonialists sought to seize the Black Hills from the original inhabitants who considered the area a sacred place. The US military used search and destroy missions and forced relocation actions against Indigenous civilians to crush native opposition (Dunbar-Ortiz, 2014, 149–153). As commander of the Seventh Cavalry, Lieutenant Colonel George Custer was tasked with coordinating and executing attacks on Indigenous communities to eliminate the native and open up resources for extractive capitalism.

George Custer was known for his rebellious and rule-breaking nature. He barely graduated from the US Military Academy at West Point, placing last in his class with a record number of demerits. Despite being a poor student, Custer proved to be a fierce soldier, serving in the Civil War and later in the Union occupation force in Texas, though he was twice court martialed for misconduct. Known for his flamboyant and vain ways, such as wearing a black velvet uniform, scenting his hair with cinnamon, and wearing a red scarf around his neck, Custer was not popular among the troops, who viewed him as narcissistic, arrogant, and tyrannical (Utley, 2001).

In 1875, President Ulysses S. Grant took action to seize control of the Black Hills, which were in Lakota territory. Following a history of continuously broken treaties on the part of the US, the Lakota and Sioux were ordered to return to their reservations away from the Black Hills. When they did not comply in the midst of winter weather and poor communication, the US commenced military action to remove the Indigenous People. As commander of the Seventh Cavalry, Custer learned of a meeting between the leaders of the Sioux, Northern Cheyenne and Arapaho peoples and attacked them at the Battle of Little Bighorn with 700 troops in 1876. Custer's twelve companies of soldiers were completely destroyed, and he was killed in the ensuing battle, which was one of the major defeats in American military history.

Much like the Charge of the Light Brigade, an ill-fated British attack on Russian forces during the Crimean War, which was memorialized by Alfred Lord Tennyson in an epic poem that emphasized the gallantry of the troops in the face of certain defeat, Custer's Last Stand was later considered to be a heroic and noble failure. Hundreds of paintings, books, and films have been devoted to constructing the valiant myth of the Battle of Little Bighorn. Supporting a monument at Little Bighorn, President Theodore Roosevelt said that Custer "has become, in a peculiar sense, the typical representative of the American regular officer who fought for the extension of our frontier" (quoted in Laas, 1994, 278). Custer, like the British Light Brigade, became a symbol of unquestioning and selfless fidelity to the settler colonial cause. The Seventh Cavalry adopted *Garryowen* as its regimental tune in 1867, and legend has it that Custer played the tune every time his soldiers began a massacre of Indigenous Peoples (Dippie, 1966). *Garryowen* may thus heard differently by settler colonialists and Indigenous Peoples and perhaps even by Irish people.

Garryowen, popular also with British, Canadian, and Australian regiments, remained a Seventh Cavalry regimental song in the twentieth century and was adopted as the official song of the US Army First Cavalry Division in 1981. It was also incorporated into the regimental crest and was used as a secret password during the Vietnam War when American troops entered 'Indian Country' when engaging with the Vietnamese. In the official story of the First Cavalry, the history of the tune is linked to the rolling green hills of Limerick, and its association with drinking is minimized. Some histories tie early versions of *Garryowen* to young rogues who drank excessively and behaved like hooligans wringing the necks of geese in their inebriated celebrations, thus showing the connection between toxic masculinity and violence from the very genesis of the song. However, the US military provides a more sedate version in their official history. The First Cavalry deemphasizes the link with Custer, writing only of his men "who rode into history," eliding any mention of the massacre of Indigenous People (First Cavalry Association, 2019). However popular the tune continues to be, is it possible to listen to *Garryowen* without the baggage of Custer? The soundtrack of *Garryowen* keeps resonating down through the generations, always in distinct tones, pitches, and contexts.

Lessons on pathways

The experience of music is profoundly physical. We embody sound by using our arms to beat drums and pursing our lips to whistle and filling our lungs to blow horns. There are deep connections between the emotion relayed by the vibrations of sound and the physical experience of movement, a topic which we take up in the next chapter. Music is a collective experience providing an emotional rhythm to create formations, marches, dances, ceremonies, and celebrations. How music is understood and interpreted depends on the relationship of the maker of the music to the culture in which it is experienced. Marching bands, for example, create a synergy between collective movement and music to build martial or competitive emotions to cheer on militaries or sports teams. Dance and movement are intimately linked with music and have sometimes been seen as a threat by authorities. In twentieth-century pop culture, Elvis Presley's hip movements and Beyoncé's twerking have been seen as expressions that could threaten the social order by inciting dangerous emotions and physical feelings and perhaps even inducing illicit thoughts. By controlling musical creativity and its embodiment, authorities have sought to shut down potentially subversive emotions and their physical expression.

Art and music can be appropriated to decontextualize and change the meaning of a piece. While all art does appropriate to some extent – by repurposing and refashioning objects, sounds, and images – appropriation can also take on colonizing aspects, especially when art is used to invoke a false sense of tradition or exoticism. Many have noted how modernist art, which arose with colonial science in the West, readily appropriated the spiritual and historical symbols of many Indigenous and Native peoples around the world. This appropriation was often a conscious act by emerging colonial powers, such as the United Kingdom, which sought to solidify power through the appropriation of symbols. Hobsbawn and Ranger (2012, 1) use the term 'invented tradition' to mean "a set of practices, normally governed by overtly or tacitly accepted rules and of a ritual or symbolic nature, which seeks to inculcate certain values and norms of behavior by repetition, which automatically implies continuity with the past." Invented traditions, therefore, often rely on the appropriation of defeated or colonized peoples' symbols to erase the meaning and significance of the conquered culture. The Iroquois eagle clutching a bundle of arrows, for example, moved from a symbol of unity in which all arrows were bound together indicating mutuality and solidarity to becoming a symbol of war on the US dollar bill.

As settler colonialism turned to nation building in the nineteenth century, music and visual art were made central parts of the project. Patriotic songs have long been used to stir emotions and loyalty to a nation. Nations have sought to consciously develop a national genre of music, often erasing or ignoring minority cultures as an attempt to homogenize and purify the nation, an entity antithetical to multiculturalism. The emphasis on patriotic music often diminishes the quality of music education because it limits the influences and ways of making music. The music of empire was translated into the vernacular for the common man. Jeffrey Richards' study of imperialism and music (2002) shows how the music of empire pervaded the dance halls, films, churches, and picnics of the United Kingdom. *Garryowen*, similarly, provides an emotional link for many Americans to the past of conquest while sustaining a sense of honor, joy, identity, and common purpose.

Nations colonize representations and sounds. National anthems are officially sanctioned songs that are said to represent the nation. They have been used to lead troops into battle and compel loyalty to a singular national identity by citizens. The gender of national anthems is almost always masculine, and the songs often evoke an eternal sense of national belonging that is exclusive and defined by blood (Sondermann, 1997). Similar to *Garryowen*, the US national anthem ("The Star-Spangled Banner") is thought to have originated as a drinking song. Patriotic marching song composer John Philip Sousa opposed the adoption of the "Star-Spangled Banner" as national anthem because of its difficult register and warlike spirit (Abril, 2012, 80). It nonetheless became the official national anthem of the United States in 1931. Music, according to Lily Hirsch (2012, 22), "reinforces territory as a symbolic language by signaling to those who belong and rejecting those who do not through an encoded system of association." The fiery national controversy over football quarterback Colin Kaepernick, who knelt during the playing the American national anthem in protest at police brutality against Black people, shows how music is marshaled to reinforce the violence and discipline of the settler colonial ideology long after nation-building is underway.

Beyond the ideology of settler colonialism, creative expression has been subject to the dynamics of extractive capitalism, making it a commodity. Art and music have thus been divided into genres and ranked in value on a scale from low to high brow, which was generally associated with colonial ideologies of race, gender, sexuality, and social class. Artistic taste uplifts certain types of creative expression as edifying, while others are disparaged as common. Classical music and opera, for example, are seen as the fine arts, while forms of music deemed 'vernacular,' such as jazz, folk, and pop, are often viewed as a less sophisticated or valuable artistic forms. European art hangs in prominent museums, while Indigenous art is often relegated to the category of 'folk' or 'primitive' craft. These ways of evaluating the worthiness of art have reinforced racialized, gendered, and class hierarchies of taste by institutionally marginalizing non-Eurocentric ways of creative expression.

Colonial music standards have often diminished and silenced or commodified and appropriated Indigenous musical expression, though Indigenous music has retained many of its subversive qualities. Hawaiian music, for example, has been a very popular genre used to market tourism, but it has also played an important role in raising Native consciousness (Franklin and Lyons, 2004). Lucrative contracts often recolonize the music of locals by corporatizing and copyrighting collective music production by inserting the logic of extractive capitalism into creative expression. Many white rock and roll stars of the 1960s built their repertoire by appropriating the sound of African American musicians who died penniless and without credit. Music in the twenty-first century has become tightly linked to corporate control. Each digital download exacts a fee and piracy is prosecuted, though the actual artists derive very little profit. After 9/11, music scholar Benjamin Robertson (2007) notes, there was greater attention to high fidelity, and music is now listened to individually on devices with headphones on which the purity of sound is highly valued. The messiness of the collective experience is increasingly removed from the intensely private and pure ways of listening to musical expression. Monetized down to the dollar, music is increasingly unprofitable for artists who have less and less contact with audiences.

Music is more commonly used as a weapon of dominance and control. It has been used by law enforcement as a means of crime prevention by discouraging loitering. Lily Hirsch describes how Australian government officials blasted Barry Manilow to drive noisy teenagers out of a parking lot. According to Hirsch (2012, 12), "the authorities effectively initiated a sonic brawl by fighting noise produced by the teens with noise controlled by the state." Music is thus weaponized to displace those deemed deviant and undesirable.

Music has played a central role in torture since the US invasion of Panama in 1989, when ousted President Manuel Noriega took refuge inside the Vatican Embassy amidst a deafening barrage of American pop music (Parker, 2019). Pieslak points out that heavy metal music was played so loudly and relentlessly during the Iraq War that one area became known as 'LalaFallujah' (Pieslak, 2009, 84). In US torture centers such as Abu Ghraib, Mosul, Bagram, and Guantanamo, music played a central role in enforcing submission and destroying the personality of the captive (Moeller and Sivak, 2012). Relentlessly playing the "I love you" song from the children's show *Barney* or heavy metal or Britney Spears at high decibel levels disorients and causes great distress to prisoners while leaving no marks (Pieslak, 2010). Why is heavy metal, for example, so prevalent in the weaponizing of American musical culture as a force of settler colonial domination? Pieslak suggests that there is a relationship between the way soldiers use the music to get pumped up for battle and how civilians and prisoners are dehumanized, thus blurring the boundaries between soldiers' excitement and the repression of prisoners. Settler colonialism and extractive capitalism thus weaponize creative expression as a tool of domination as well as alienation and estrangement.

Visual art as colonizer

Michael shares a story

Imagine for a moment that you are a descendant of a people who were the first to arrive and settle in a land, long before any other group could even fathom that such a place even existed. Your people ventured forth through hardships, some walking across great divides of land, others navigating great bodies of water, and others crossing massive ice sheets during some of the most inclement weather. When they arrived, they claimed, settled, and occupied these places and lived here for tens of thousands of years – probably even longer than that. In fact, many of you believe that your people have always resided here, and their origin stories tell of how you emerged from these lands, mountains, waters, jungles, and deserts, and have a strong, abiding connection and love for all these places.

Over the course of your history, you survived and thrived during drastic climate changes, droughts, starvation, and war. Your people settled and changed the landscape. In some places, you marked them with amazing structures, cities, and towns. Some residences were carved into cliffs, some were built along the rivers and oceans, and some found refuge and a way of living that was deep within jungles or in arid, harsh deserts. Others were erected in seemingly impossible locations, high among the clouds in ancient mountains, some on frozen lands or deep within areas of hot humid swamps with little land to support them. Your people left many signs of their presence that have been here for thousands and thousands of years. Some are still visible today: earthen mounds and temples, pyramids, petroglyph carvings on rocks, ancient medicine wheels, burial grounds, trading routes, and effigies carved out of rock and wood and fashioned into totem poles. Every now and then you visit these places, and it may bring a tear or feelings of awe as your genetic memory recalls why your people occupied, visited, and consecrated these areas. In other places, your people left the lands and waters in their original state, using them as natural pharmacies, markets for hunting and gathering, places of spiritual sanctuary, or treading lightly in those areas that were owned and occupied by the animals or spirit guardians.

Now, imagine that a new people arrive, people unlike any you've ever seen before. They are ill-equipped to survive in your territory, so some of your people offer them what they need to survive. The newcomers are friendly at first, but soon you learn that they believe that you and your people are not equal to them and are not worthy of respect. You learn that they hold a belief that a divine being that they call god has endowed them with the power and responsibility to eliminate you or make you become like them. Soon they condemn you for how you look, believe, speak, live, and behave. They label your people 'savages' and 'heathens' and call your culture 'primitive.' They say that their god has ordered them to take your lands, destroy your civilizations, and wipe you out if you do not become like them.

They continue to arrive, in wave after wave, and begin to move into your lands without your permission and invade with forceful violence. When you resist their encroachment, they kill you. In one of their most sacred documents that they call their 'Declaration of Independence,' in order to further their cause and justify their theft of your territories and killing of your peoples, they refer to your people as "merciless Indian savages."

Now, imagine that they begin a more systematic and coordinated effort to eliminate everyone like you. They enslave your people, steal your children, and rape and sex traffic the women; they kill your intellectuals, imprison your spiritual leaders, and deny you of anything that enables you to resist. They spread their foreign diseases among you, sometimes accidently, other times deliberately, and millions of you are killed off. Some of them offer bounties for your bloody scalp; it doesn't matter if you are a child, a woman, or an elder. They burn your towns, plunder your resources, and pillage your sacred sites; they destroy your food supplies, and they raze your monuments and remove you from your lands – if they don't kill you first. And then, when your numbers have diminished and you can no longer resist, they round you up and relocate you to the most barren lands, where they force you to live. They call them reservations, rancherias, or reserves. Finally, they commence a long campaign of teaching generation after generation about the supremacy of their people and the inferiority of you and your people. This belief gets deeply embedded in their laws, history, education, religion, politics, and economies. Soon you are forgotten . . . and they have achieved the white nationalism they so desired.

In the future, they name their sports teams after you, mocking your culture with distorted racist images of your people and with words such as 'savages' and 'redskins.' When your descendants protest, they laugh at you and say that it's an honor be called a redskin, or that it is freedom of speech, or you need to get over the past, or that they are tired of your political correctness. Since they destroyed your history and promoted only theirs, they have history on their side. Brilliant. When they are questioned about their conquest of your people, they can say it was for a good reason – that they were worthy, white, more intelligent and civilized than your people, which reinforces their white supremacy. In their generosity, they name few military weapons, streets, bridges, roads, and landscapes after some of your tribes; some of them they say represent your bravery, while others mock you.

Since its inception, the United States of America has imagined and marketed itself as the world's greatest democracy, the beacon of hope for the rest of the world, a "shining city on the hill," and the greatest nation on earth, all the while ignoring its invasion of these lands and its genocidal history, wherein most of Indigenous population was killed off and almost all of the lands, waters, and resources were forcibly taken by invading settlers. Scholars today argue whether or not what really happened to the Indigenous Peoples in the Americas can be regarded as genocide. Many say no. But what if this admission of invasion, white supremacy, and genocide that can be dismissed in the written text is instead found in artwork, in a painting called *American Progress*, otherwise known as *Manifest Destiny*. The artist John Gast painted this picture in 1876 as a travelogue to encourage white settlers to travel, sightsee, and settle in the West. Is this picture proof enough of genocide? Let's see.

What is the first thing that you see as you look at this picture? If you are like most, it is the luminous woman in the center of the painting. She is floating above the earth as if she has the magical powers of levitation. In her overemphasized body posture, she is leaning forward with her right leg protruding from her gown, bent in a running position, almost as if she is sprinting toward her destiny. She looks like an angelic, divine being, doesn't she – with all that long wavy blonde hair and flowing gown? And she is so white. Her skin, her aura, and long flowing dress are all so white. What does it mean to be white? Some synonyms of the color white in *Merriam-Webster Dictionary* include *lacking an addition of color* as in unstained or uncolored, as opposed to "colored people" or "people of color;" *not causing or being capable of causing injury or hurt* as in innocent, harmless, and trustworthy; and finally, *free from sin* as innocent, pure, moral, and blameless. Who wouldn't want to be white?

If you look closely, you can see that she is wearing the 'the star of the empire,' on her forehead, a symbol of American imperialism, a policy of extending and imposing the power and authority of the United States over other territories and peoples through economic, political, and social dominance. And, when you compare the color or tint of the sky and clouds behind and in front of her, you realize that the artist wanted to you see that she is bringing forth the light of civilization to chase away the primitive darkness before her. It's a very clever technique that we may not even consciously notice if it isn't pointed out.

A book is tucked tightly under right arm. What is the book? A lot of people, at first glance, think it is the Christian Bible. But I always like to say it is text more powerful and influential than that. It's a schoolbook that recounts the history and greatness of this nation's leaders, its amazing progress, exceptionalism, and civilization. By the way, Bibles are not compulsory reading for schoolchildren, but schoolbooks are. She is also holding and stringing along a telegraph cable. Can you see the telegraph poles behind her? She is establishing a transcontinental communication network between the eastern and western United States that will provide a form of high-speed (compared to the pony express) communication between the east and west coasts.

In the far-lower right, there are farmers who are plowing fields behind a pair of oxen. When I look at what they are doing, I can't help think of how much destruction of Indigenous People's wild prairie lands, waters, wild medicines, and insect and animal habitat occurred due to the early unsustainable farming practices of American farmers. Even with sustainable practices today, farming continues to use deadly, toxic 'weedkillers' like Monsanto's Roundup (main ingredient, glyphosate), which has been proven to kill human cells and cause birth defects and cancer. For years, on my reservation and throughout the United States, settler farming and ranching practices used a deadly pesticide called DDT (dichlorodiphenyltrichloroethane), which had devastating impacts on the health of the environment, animals, and humans.

Just a bit in front of the farmers are the mining prospectors and explorers, heading west to find fame and fortune. In the past and in the present, miners and mining, like so many other settlers and settler activities, have often been regarded as the epitome of evil by Indigenous Peoples. In the years of the California genocide, miners, settlers, and citizen militias murdered and kidnapped enslaved Indigenous Peoples and forced them off their lands. California, like so many other places in the United States, can be considered killing fields, where thousands of Indigenous Peoples were murdered. How high was the death toll? Demographers estimate that in the 1760s, there were as many as 300,000 California natives. By 1900, only 16,000 remained. As many as 17,000 were murdered during the California gold rush, many of them taken prisoner and used as slave labor, dying from disease, starvation, and abuse. In front of Columbia, we see the trains, steamships, covered wagons, and stagecoaches speeding to the west. From the trains, passengers, hunters, and military soldiers routinely shot and killed thousands and thousands of buffalo that were near the train tracks. American military General William Sherman, who had spent many years carrying out war against Indigenous Peoples of the Plains, held a deep contempt for them. To eliminate them, he knew that the buffalo had to be eradicated. He responded by calling on the US Army to do their part: "Let them kill, skin, and sell until the buffalo is exterminated, as it is the only way to bring lasting peace and allow civilization to advance" (quoted in Grygiel, 2018, 206)

The last groups in the picture that can be seen in the dim light are the Indians, wolves, buffalo, and grizzly bears. They are positioned in front of Columbia, looking up and back at her, and it appears that they are running in fear for their lives. They are the predators, the savages, the beasts that must be targeted for elimination so white settler civilization can emerge and manifest. Wolves once populated much of North America but were drastically reduced in number by settlers since they felt they posed a risk to humans, their livestock, pets, and the game animals they hunted. Today, wolves remain on the endangered list but are slowly making a comeback. Grizzly bears followed much of the same fate as wolves and also ended up listed as a "threatened" species on the US Endangered Species Act.

Finally, but not surprisingly, Indigenous Peoples in the United States followed the same trajectory as the wolves, buffalo, and bears after meeting European and American settlers: invasion, death, removal, and near extinction. Wars, enslavement, disease, and campaigns of neglect, broken promises, and genocide drastically reduced the populations of Indigenous Peoples in the Americas. In many instances, the abuse and persecution that Indigenous Peoples experienced at the hands of settler society is unimaginable, as Indigenous historian Donald Fixico (2019), one the nation's pre-imminent American Indian scholars, has long documented.

So, who is this woman in the picture that leads the vanguard of manifest destiny, settler colonialism, and genocide? Her name is Columbia. At one time she was considered to be the historical name for the United States. She was regarded as the female counterpart to Christopher Columbus, the historical figure credited with "discovering" America, but who has been more recently recognized as the individual responsible for launching the brutal European and American invasion of the Americas. Columbia was invented by Americans to denote their patriotism and is associated with their idea of being a world power. After World War II, she was replaced by Lady Liberty, a goddess-like female personification of the United States, but the most famous image of Columbia was created by American painter John Gast.

Many people have associated her with the doctrine of Manifest Destiny, the belief that Americans were destined and divinely inspired (by God) to settle the entire United States from East Coast to West. Manifest Destiny meant that Americans must bring their ideas of commerce, education, religion, democracy, and civilization to all areas unsettled by white people. Classic settler colonialism is about eliminating the native and dispossessing them of their lives, lands, waters, forests, culture, resources, and rights, often using war and murder, deliberately spreading diseases, such as smallpox, or hunting out all of the game so Indigenous Peoples would starve, or making and breaking deals (treaties never meant to be honored by settlers) with Indigenous Peoples to get the job done. To the land- and resource-hungry Americans, Indigenous Peoples were not civilized, as we can see in John Gast's picture. They were savages who knew nothing of God and had no laws, morality, or industry. Again, not too much different than the buffalo, grizzly bear, or wolves. Their communal ways of sharing the land, loyalty to the community, and respect for all of nature were considered to be primitive, backward, and barely, if at all, human attributes. Of course, the Americans considered themselves to be God's chosen people, endowed with the responsibility to civilize Indigenous Peoples, which is why Gast's picture called *American Progress* makes so much sense for settlers.

If just for a moment we isolate Columbus from his sister Columbia, we can see that many Americans continue to overlook, ignore, and trivialize the impact that Columbus had on Indigenous Peoples and continue to celebrate the Italian's 'discovery' as a hallmark of human progress and civilization. On October 16, 2019, when asked about the ongoing controversy about Columbus Day during a press conference at the White House, President Donald Trump responded, "To me it will always be called Columbus Day. Some people don't like that, I do." On the other hand, numerous Indigenous Peoples and settler allies in the Western Hemisphere continue to oppose and protest the celebration of Columbus Day, recognizing the suffering, death, and abuse that he brought on his mission of discovery. It has taken many years of protest and education to offset the damage and lies of the Columbia legacy.

Most people within and beyond the borders of the United States have never heard of Columbia as she been described in this narrative, probably because she is the softer side of white supremacy, and she is a painting of the past, an artifact of colonialism and American imperialism that has long passed into the sphere of postcolonial oblivion. And we don't know her because she doesn't directly bloody her hands with conquest. Instead she inspires, brings the light to expose the enemies, and provides the means for this to happen. While we may think the days of Columbia have long passed, her name lives on by way of cities, states, countries, products, and Hollywood movies. She will always be with us. And if you ever want to see the new and improved Columbia, thinner, more fit, with skin and hair that is just a bit darker, you can see her at the very opening of many Hollywood movies.

So, imagine for a moment that you are the descendant of the first peoples to arrive and settle in this land. And now you are looking up at this picture titled *American Progress*, depicting a very white woman who is floating above you, whose light enabled the genocide of your ancestors.

More lessons on pathways

The deep structures of settler colonialism, militarism, and white privilege have been powerful drivers of creative taste through academia and artistic production industries. Yet schooling is perhaps the primary means of inculcating ideas of beauty, worthiness, and visibility through the colonial curriculum. Frantz Fanon (1970), the renowned Martinican psychiatrist, wrote of the complex ways that the superiority of whiteness was instilled in children of color. In describing how Black children in French-speaking areas of the Caribbean repeated every morning at school: "We are the children of the fair-haired Gauls," Fanon (1963) underlined the how school erased ancestry and place. Art has served an important colonizing purpose by teaching children to admire certain kinds of representations and sounds as superior while disparaging others as inferior, as we can see in Michael's story of Columbia in which the superiority of the white woman leading progress exerts dominion over the dark Indigenous subjects.

By restricting the validity of artistic subjects and expression, many feel alienation and estrangement from authentic expression and indeed themselves. Like the silencing effect of trauma, we are diminished when the act of creative expression is stolen from us through the enforcement of artistic standards and taste. In the landmark *Brown v. Board of Education* ruling in the US Supreme Court in 1954, judges cited the famous Clark study of dolls to be compelling evidence of how images of racism have a deleterious impact on the self-esteem of children (Loder-Jackson, Christiansen, and Kelly, 2016). In the Clark study, which considered the psychological impact of racial segregation, children between the ages of three and seven years old were asked to identify the races and characteristics of four baby dolls. The majority of children identified the white dolls as the prettiest with the most positive social and physical characteristics. In writing about his practice with colonized subjects, Frantz Fanon (1963) pointed out the personal impact of the erasure of Indigenous identities. The systemic dispossession of Indigenous and colonized peoples from their land and cultures has produced historical trauma that, as we noted in Chapter 3, reverberates on personal, community, and structural levels down the generations as destructive emotions, dysfunctional behaviors, and debilitating actions.

The structures and ideologies of settler colonialism alienate us from one another and estrange us from our own ways of expression by introducing the logic of extractive capitalism and commodification into the deepest parts of our consciousness and soul. How do we decolonize our relationship to playing and listening to music, making and looking at art, and experiencing creative expression when our orientation to art and music has become so deeply entangled with the ongoing structures of settler colonialism? How do we open up to new understandings and orientations towards creative expression that heal rather than oppress? Creative expression has a healing force if liberated to be the gift that it is. These are some of the questions that emerge as we consider our relationship to creative expression in a settler colonial world of extractive capitalism.

Decolonized creative expression enacts resistance to the epistemic colonization that privileges Western aesthetics. As Burke Stanton notes (2018, 6): "Epistemic colonization is . . . a framework for understanding a decolonization of music, invites us to ponder the making of the musical worlds we inhabit and how we understand them." Similarly, as Laura E. Pérez richly documents in *Chicana Art: The Politics of Spiritual and Aesthetic Altarities* (2007), how we perceive what art is reflects our relationship to coloniality. In opening up the visual landscape of Chicana altars embedded in place, gender, and history, Pérez maps a terrain largely unseen by mainstream art critics. The use of ofrendas and murals, especially during important events like the Day of the Dead, decolonizes mourning and spirituality, grounding Chicano and Latinx communities in precolonial ancient knowledge and imagery. Long disregarded by the art world as mundane folk art, nowadays many Mexican-American, Chicano, and Latinx communities struggle with settler colonial commercial attempts to appropriate and recolonize Indigenous social imaginaries for profit.

Cultural policy and art museums serve important public functions. Funded by taxpayers, these cultural institutions collect artifacts and art to display as a means of interpreting the notion of 'heritage' and culture to the masses (Fladmark, 2000). Cultural policies have institutionalized the norms and boundaries of the national and the artistic through museum evaluations that erase queerness and dehumanize people of color. In recent years, there has been greater critique of many objects stolen from colonized lands resting in Western museums.

The *Apeshit* video by Beyoncé and Jay-Z presents a thickly visual exploration of settler colonial art consumption. Filmed in the center of Western art culture, the Louvre, Beyoncé and Jay-Z meander through room after room of white subjects. They look at the *Mona Lisa*, the most famous Renaissance painting by Leonardo da Vinci, in the eye as equals. Beyoncé asserts the centrality of Black female sensuality in a context that has often dehumanized or objectified it (Silberstein, 2019). The video ends with Marie Benoist's *Portrait d'une négresse*, one of the few paintings of a free Black person. Throughout the video, Beyoncé brings an assertion of female power in the midst of settler colonial, white, patriarchal art. It represents a takeover of white space and assertion of Black beauty and worthiness in the heart of the European artworld.

The *Apeshit* video as well as the altars and ofrendas described by Pérez model ways of talking back to colonized standards of beauty, worthiness, and creative expression. Far from being passive receptacles of settler colonial aesthetic standards, various and diverse artists are working to challenge the long dominance of settler colonial standards, reasserting the validity of ancient Indigenous forms of creative expression and faced firmly towards a decolonized future.

Creative expression as integrative social work practice

Psychology and social work have a long tradition of using art, music, and other forms of creative expression. There has been a vast amount of research into creative expression and how it contributes to mental health (e.g., Forgeard, Mecklenburg, Lacasse, and Jayawickreme, 2014; Frantz, 2016). Here, we will briefly highlight how the use of the arts as healing emerged with changing views of working with people with mental health issues. The field of arts and healing is enormous and diverse, far larger than we could capture in this small section. Hence, our goal is to illustrate how creative expression has been incorporated into the mainstream of integrative social work practice and to explore decolonizing pathways of creative expression. We end the chapter with a story from Michael about the healing role of music in his family.

With the rise of the industrial capitalism in the modern settler colonial world, people with mental health issues were increasingly isolated into huge asylums, which proliferated throughout the Western world in the 1800s. While mental illness was often seen as a form of possession by the devil in medieval times, the modern era brought a more medicalized and industrialized approach to mental health. Asylums used coercion, moral blame, and stigma to label and confine non-conforming members of industrial capitalist settler colonial societies. Many institutions kept inmates occupied with labor as a means to produce resources to help cover the costs of expensive institutionalization. In keeping with the Protestant work ethic, business was viewed as a moral virtue. Hence approaches to mental health treatment in the nineteenth century often used work as punishment, moral therapy, and a medical regimen (Ernst, 2018). Industrial societies in general required more labor than people had previously performed with working hours estimated to increase by 20% (Voth, 1997). The rise of workhouses and asylums was thus directly tied with the punitive and moralistic code of the new ethics of unceasing labor emerging under capitalism (Foucault, 1977).

In the nineteenth century, notions of mental health long embedded in the exclusionary institution of the asylum were shifting with the internalization of structural capitalist and settler colonial relations. Emerging 'psychological individualism' saw people as autonomously responsible for their mental states. As psychologist Craig Haney (1982, 198) notes,

> the ideology of individualism also may have served another function – that of easing the psychological strains imposed by an increasingly fluid and diverse society. Status-bound and traditional societies not only impose real

limitations on their members but also provide some measure of security, at least for *certain* segments of the society. Remove the limits and undermine stability – proceed from status to contract – and anxiety as well as freedom results for some.

New ways of living under settler colonial extractive capitalism drove certain kinds of anxiety and mental health disorders because of the intrinsic insecurity of contingent relationships.

Straddling the divide between physiological and psychological medical etiology, early psychiatry embraced talk therapy, dreamwork, and exploring the mind as loci of healing. Sigmund Freud and Carl Jung explored the role that the unconscious plays in our actions and thoughts. Psychiatry emerged as art movements like Impressionism and Expressionism also challenged conventional notions of realism by portraying inner states of mind on the canvas. Many early psychiatrists showed great interest in the artwork of mental asylum residents and wanted to explore whether there was a link between madness and creativity. Hans Prinzkampf, a Viennese psychiatrist and art historian, explored the art of mental patients not simply as reflections of pathology but also as an aesthetic work of art (Cohen, 2017). Moreover, emerging modalities helped shift ways of working with psychological distress from that of sin, punishment, and shame towards active engagement with mental illness through talk and creative expression.

The roots of art and creative crafts in social work practice can be traced back to the Belle Époque, or the historical period in Western Europe right before the First World War. The British Arts and Crafts Movement sought to preserve the unique craftsmanship of the applied arts despite growing industrialization and standardization by practicing and restoring traditional handiwork. Early occupational therapy at the turn of the century worked with chronically ill patients by facilitating arts and crafts (Levine, 1987). Many physicians also recognized the therapeutic value of creating and making, which became a prominent feature of treatment in American state hospitals.

Psychoanalysts in the United States, such as Margaret Naumberg and Edith Kramer, were important drivers of the development of the professional field of art therapy in the 1940s, a field which also had deep roots in occupational therapy. Naumberg and Kramer saw art as more than revealing unconscious states; rather, they viewed creating itself as healing (Brooke, 2006). All of these shifts in ways of thinking and valuing the role of how we express feelings through creativity and artistic forms opened possibilities for their inclusion in therapeutic practice. Edward Adamson, for example, pioneered the use of art as a therapeutic modality with chronic patients in mental health institutions in the United Kingdom (O'Flynn, 2011). He also collected and arranged showings of patients' art to educate the public. As teaching artist Rachel Cohen (2017, 101) observes: "It is likely due to the fact that these early practitioners held identities as artists and were engaged with modern art forms that led them to prioritize making over analyzing."

During the Great Depression, the Works Progress Administration (WPA) Federal Art Project funded artists to create art in public places throughout the United States. At Bellevue Hospital, a mental health institution in New York, WPA mural painters engaged with patients and occupational therapy. Space is transformed by art, which is why hospitals and other institutions have been increasingly turning to artistic collaborate to develop visually healing spaces. Some studies even suggest that interacting with art can boost the immune system by reducing inflammation (Stuckey and Nobel, 2010). Visual art enhances the mind-body connection and promotes healing.

Creative expression thus became seen as a means to uncover the unconscious as well as connecting to others as healing process. Art therapy has emerged as a professional specialty with links to a multitude of fields, including early education, psychotherapy, social work, counseling, and gerontology, and has been viewed as a useful intervention in many state institutions (Davidow, 2018). Art psychotherapies have supported people living with cancer to express their daily struggles. Emphasizing the need for the establishment of a therapeutic relationship before starting art therapy, Schiltz and Zimoch (2017, 52) discuss how art helps cancer patients develop the "imaginary and symbolic elaboration" of conflicts and difficulties. It is effective because it is not just 'talking' but also 'doing.' Encouraging artistic creativity has been seen an important means for patients to explore their own unconscious and express thoughts and feelings.

While these highlights of the emergence of art therapy as a mainstream therapeutic practice have touched on many of the widely perceived professional pioneers who developed the field, it is important to underline the significance of decolonized practice of creative expression as healing. Rachel Cohen (2017), for example, writes of artist-attendants who connected with patients in mental institutions as fellow artists. Nicole Rangel (2016) discusses decolonizing healing as embracing the collectivity of ancestral lineage, relationality, and the principle of love. By firmly centering healing as connection, Rangel's focuses on poetry as a method of decolonized healing. Lu and Yuen (2012) talk about a project called 'Journey Women' in which Aboriginal women created body maps of the impact of colonial violence on themselves. Healing through creative expression requires an epistemic shift that allows us, as discussed in the previous section, to ponder the creative worlds we live in and reorient our ways of expressing ourselves.

Michael's story

Some years ago, my grandfather, Joe Reed, told me that our music, songs, and some of our ceremonies originally came to us from dreams, visions, spirits, insects, birds, and other animals. He said that the waters, winds, blowing grasses, stars, and other forms of life also influenced our music. Songs and dances were part of our everyday life. They were performed to acknowledge the changing of the seasons, to send young men to war or to celebrate peace, to help send someone along on their spirit journey after they had passed, and to celebrate the birth of a child or perform the yearly public blessing of the children. Some societies performed songs and dances such as the buffalo or bear dance to acknowledge the strong healing power of these animals which were important when healers were performing traditional doctoring. Songs were an important feature of one's identity. Many individuals were given their own personal song by prominent elders or spiritual leaders, that described who they were as they grew to adulthood and elder status, often describing and praising their laudable traits and behaviors.

The songs of the Arikara are sung in the either cultural language or through the use of vocables, which refers to singing through vocal expressions without words. Singing vocables might be best compared to singing notes on a musical scale without using words. Vocables can sound like a person imitating the sounds and notes of an instrument. In the world of jazz, this is known as scat singing. Vocables were also used to imitate the sounds of animals, birds, thunders, rain, winds, and spirits. The Sámi, Indigenous Peoples from Finland, Norway, and Sweden, use a vocable technique called joiking and the vocable style of the Inuit and Mongolian peoples is known as throat singing.

I come from a family of musicians that extends back many generations. My father's grandfather Yellow Bird, whom I mentioned earlier, was known as a very special and talented ceremonial singer. One of my father's sisters was a very accomplished singer who sang contemporary religious songs and one grandmother was a trained classical pianist. All fifteen of my brothers and sisters at one time played a woodwind, brass, or string instrument, and a few were vocal performers who won important formal school competitions and community talent shows. One of my favorite stories of how traditional Arikara music was used as prayer and a daily celebration of life in my family comes from my father.

When my father was a young boy he lived with his grandfather, Plenty Fox. Grandpa Plenty Fox was a traditional Arikara elder who spoke only the Arikara language and clung tightly to our cultural ceremonies and traditions. Although he understood English, he detested it and refused to speak it, citing its inability to describe the full humanity of the Arikara world.

Not long ago, during the summertime, the natural prairie landscape on our reservation was carpeted by beautiful wildflowers, short grasses, scrub trees that produce wild berries, and hills that reflect earth tone colors such as ochre, sienna, and umber. Our lands are home to little creatures such as damsel flies, stink bugs, ground beetles, crickets, horned toads, and rattlesnakes that hum, buzz, chirp, and rattle continuously throughout the day and night. Larger animals like mule and whitetail deer, badgers, moose, elk, mountain lions, porcupines, and prairie dogs are also familiar residents. During his time with Grandpa Plenty Fox, my father said that grandpa told him that all the life that we see, whether plants, insects, birds, earth, or animals, all have their own way of praying, their own ceremonies, and their own way of dancing and singing. He said that all creatures love their own children and their people, but just like humans, they sometimes they experience hardships or have times that they don't get along with each other. In the present day, this natural diversity of life has been greatly diminished by the excessive farming practices of settlers that live on or near the reservation and the development of oil fields throughout our territory.

The world that my grandfather Plenty Fox grew up in was steeped in traditional ancient ceremonies, music, dances, and the honoring and use of sacred bundles that chronicled our tribe's long, arduous spiritual journey. My father was born on the edge of these times. Daily life for our people was a constant stream of prayer and ceremony, interspersed with gender-specific roles and recreational activities that promoted unity and enjoyment. In the village, both secular and sacred women and men's societies, venerated by the tribe, engaged in special ritual practices, dances, songs, and prayers that acknowledged the ancestors, all forms of life, and the people's place in the world. Rather than doing a google search for answers, our people sought wisdom and protection from the spirits and ancestors that resided in the four quarters (semi-cardinal directions) of Mother Earth.

For Grandpa Plenty Fox everyday was a prayer, a song, and a ritual which began every morning when he awoke. Before he let his feet touch the earth, while he was still lying in bed, he would sing an Arikara blessing song, thanking the Creator for another day of life and asking for help for the people so that they may live good lives and the tribe might prosper. His song included an acknowledgement to the northeast direction for his rest and to the Night for the teachings he derived from his dreams. When he finished his first song of the day, he would sit in silence at the edge of his bed in deep meditative prayer. Soon he called to my father, telling him it was time to go outside and sing to the Sunrise. As they stood outside, Grandpa Plenty Fox would begin rhythmically shaking his gourd rattle as he began singing to the first light of morning.

Grandpa had two horses in a corral next to his house and three dogs that lived under the house. When he started singing his song, the horses would immediately trot to the fence to listen, while the dogs would come out from under the house and sit side by side next to my father, who was standing next to Grandpa Plenty Fox. Occasionally, the dogs and my father would exchange glances during the singing, but none of them would look at Grandpa. As if on cue, during certain phrases or tones in the music, the dogs would close their eyes and start howling in the direction of the rising sun. Sometimes my Grandpa would wipe tears from his eyes as he sang in humility before all of creation.

When the singing was finished, the dogs would be fed, and Grandpa and my father would go inside for breakfast. As the food was prepared, Grandpa would begin speaking Arikara to the food as if it could understand him. After he finished talking to it, he would begin singing to the spirits of the different foods. My father would watch and quietly sing along. My father said sometimes it took a long time before we were able to eat. After breakfast, Grandpa Plenty Fox would sing another blessing song in thanks for the meal.

My father said that whenever Grandpa Plenty Fox and he had to travel somewhere, they used a team of horses that pulled them in a buckboard wagon. As they rode along, Grandpa would tell stories about all of the plants, flowers, and creatures they encountered along the way. He explained how they came about and what they represented to the people; even the lands, hills, and waters had their own stories and songs. Dad said sometimes they would travel for long distances without speaking and then, all of sudden, Grandpa would begin singing or say a long, beautiful prayer. At the end of the long day as my father lay in his bed he would fall asleep listening to Grandpa Plenty Fox singing a prayer song or a going away song, maybe in preparation for his journey to the spirit world.

Years later, long after Grandpa Plenty Fox passed into the spirit world, my father formed or played with a number of bands that performed jazz, big band, polka, and country and western dance music. He became a well-known local jazz musician on and off our reservation and was locally famous for his singing and trumpet and tenor and alto saxophone playing at local dance clubs and at private or community events. Every once in while he sang traditional tribal songs with local drummers, but only when he was asked. Towards the end of his life, he maintained his drive to play music and often 'sat in' with my rock 'n roll band that I performed with in the 1970s and 1980s. There is only one time that I can recall when he sang a song he learned from Grandpa Plenty Fox. As he sang, he would sometimes pause to remember the words. After he finished singing, he had a puzzled, faraway look on his face. He sat for a moment longer and then without saying another word, he got up and went outside and got in his car and drove away. I can still see his car's red taillights disappearing into the night and hear him playing his saxophone and singing Grandpa Plenty Fox's song.

References

Abril, C. 2012. A National Anthem. In *Patriotism and Nationalism in Music Education*, edited by David G. Hebert and Alexandra Kertz-Welzel. Farnham, Surrey and Burlington, VT: Ashgate.

Beşe, A. 2012. Music as an Expression of Cultural Identity: August Wilson's Dramatic Reflections of African-American Art. *Interstudia (Revista Centrului Interdisciplinar de Studiu al Formelor Discursive Contemporane Interstud)*, 11(1): 15–29.

Brooke, S. L. 2006. *Creative Arts Therapies Manual: A Guide to the History, Theoretical Approaches, Assessment, and Work with Special Populations of Art, Play, Dance, Music, Drama, and Poetry Therapies*. Springfield, IL: Charles C Thomas Publishers.

Cohen, R. 2017. *Outsider Art and Art Therapy: Shared Histories, Current Issues and Future Identities*. London: Jessica Kingsley Publishers.

Cseh, G. M., Phillips, L. H., and Pearson, D. G. 2015, Flow, Affect and Visual Creativity. *Cognition & Emotion*, 29(2): 281–291.

Davidow, J. 2018. Art Therapy, Occupational Therapy, and American Modernism. *American Art*, 32(2): 80–99.

Dippie, B. W. 1966. Bards of the Little Big Horn. *Western American Literature*, 1(3): 175–195.

Dunbar-Ortiz, R. 2014. *An Indigenous Peoples' History of the United States*. Old Saybrook, CT: Tantor Media.

Ernst, W. 2018. The Role of Work in Psychiatry: Historical Reflections. *Indian Journal of Psychiatry*, 60(Suppl 2): S248–S252.

Fanon, F. 1963. *The Wretched of the Earth*. New York: Grove Press.

Fanon, F. 1970. *Black Skin, White Masks*. London: Paladin.

First Cavalry Association. 2019. Accessed 3 April 2020 at https://1cda.org/history/garryowen.

Fixico, D. L. 2019. Re-imagining Race and Ethnicity in the American West in the Twenty-first Century. *Western Historical Quarterly*, 50(1): 1–15.

Fladmark, J. M. 2000. *Heritage and Museums: Shaping National Identity*. Shaftesbury: Donhead.

Forgeard, M., Mecklenburg, A., Lacasse, J., and Jayawickreme, E. 2014. *Bringing the Whole Universe to Order: Creativity, Healing, and Posttraumatic Growth*. Cambridge: Cambridge University Press.

Foucault, M. 1977. *Discipline and Punish: The Birth of the Prison*. London: Penguin Books.

Franklin, C., and Lyons, L. 2004. Remixing Hybridity: Globalization, Native Resistance, and Cultural Production in Hawai'i. *American Studies*, 45(3): 49.

Frantz, G. 2016. Creativity and Healing. *Psychological Perspectives*, 59(2): 242–251.

Gleason, B. P. 2015. Military Music in the United States: A Historical Examination of Performance and Training. *Music Educators Journal*, 101(3): 37–46.

Grygiel, J. J. 2018. *Return of the Barbarians: Confronting Non-state Actors From Ancient Rome to the Present*. Cambridge: Cambridge University Press.

Haney, C. 1982. Criminal Justice and the Nineteenth – Century Paradigm: The Triumph of Psychological Individualism in the "Formative Era". *Law and Human Behavior*, 6(3–4): 191–235.

Harrington, D. M. 2018. On the Usefulness of "Value" in the Definition of Creativity: A Commentary. *Creativity Research Journal*, 30(1): 118–121.

Hirsch, L. E. 2012. *Music in American Crime Prevention and Punishment*. Ann Arbor: University of Michigan Press.

Hobsbawn, E., and Ranger, T. (eds.). 2012. *The Invention of Tradition*. Cambridge: Cambridge University Press.

Laas, V. J. 1994. Elizabeth Bacon Custer and the Making of a Myth (Review). *Civil War History*, 40(2): 167–168.

Levine, R. 1987. The Influence of the Arts-and-Crafts Movement on the Professional Status of Occupational Therapy. *The American Journal of Occupational Therapy*, 41(4): 248–254.

Loder-Jackson, T. L., Christensen, L. M., and Kelly, H. 2016. Unearthing and Bequeathing Black Feminist Legacies of Brown to a New Generation of Women and Girls. *The Journal of Negro Education*, 85(3): 199–211. https://doi.org/10.7709/jnegroeducation.85.3.0199.

Lu, L., and Yuen, F. 2012. Journey Women: Art Therapy in a Decolonizing Framework of Practice. *The Arts in Psychotherapy*, 39(3): 192–200.

Moeller, M. M., and Sivak, A. 2012. Fuck Your God in the Disco: Music, Torture, and the Divine at Guantánamo. *Radical Philosophy Review (Philosophy Documentation Center)*, 15(1): 127–144.

O'Flynn, D. 2011. Art as Healing: Edward Adamson. *Raw Vision*, 72, 46–53.

Parker, J. E. K. 2019. Sonic Lawfare: On the Jurisprudence of Weaponised Sound. *Sound Studies*, 5(1): 72–96.

Perez, L. E. 2007. *Chicana Art: The Politics of Spiritual and Aesthetic Altarities*. Berkeley: University of California.

Pieslak, J. 2010. Cranking up the Volume: Music as a Tool of Torture. *Global Dialogue (Online)*, 12(1): 1–11.

Pieslak, J. R. 2009. *Sound Targets: American Soldiers and Music in the Iraq War*. Bloomington: Indiana University Press.

Rangel, N. 2016. An Examination of Poetry for the People: A Decolonizing Holistic Approach to Arts Education. *Educational Studies*, 52(6): 536–551.

Richards, J. 2002. *Imperialism and Music: Britain, 1876–1953*. Manchester: Manchester University Press.

Robertson, B. 2007. Music, Terrorism, Response: The Conditioning Logic of Code and Networks. In *Music in the Post-9/11 World*, edited by Jonathan Ritter and J. Martin Daughtry, 31–42. New York: Routledge.

Schiltz, L., and Zimoch, A. 2017. Using Arts Psychotherapy in Psycho-Oncology as a Means of Coping with Stress and Anxiety. *Archives of Psychiatry & Psychotherapy*, 19(1): 47–55.

Silberstein, E. 2019. "Have You Ever Seen the Crowd Goin' Apeshit?": Disrupting Representations of Animalistic Black Femininity in the French Imaginary. *Humanities*, 8(3): 135.

Sondermann, K. 1997. Reading Politically: National Anthems as Textual Icon. In *Interpreting the Political: New Methodologies*, edited by Terrell Carver and Matti Hyvarinen. Abingdon: Routledge.

Stalinski, S. M., and Schellenberg, E. G. 2012. Music Cognition: A Developmental Perspective. *Topics in Cognitive Science*, 4(4): 485–497.

Stanton, B. 2018. Musicking in the Borders Toward Decolonizing Methodologies. *Philosophy of Music Education Review*, 26(1): 4–23.

Stuckey, H. L., and Nobel, J. 2010. The Connection Between Art, Healing, and Public Health: A Review of Current Literature. *American Journal of Public Health*, 100(2): 254.

Thyssen, G., and Grosvenor, I. 2019. Learning to Make Sense: Interdisciplinary Perspectives on Sensory Education and Embodied Enculturation. *The Senses and Society*, 14(2): 119–130.

Utley, R. M. 2001. *Cavalier in Buckskin: George Armstrong Custer and the Western Military Frontier*. Norman: University of Oklahoma Press.

Voth, H. J. 1997. *Time and Work in Eighteenth-Century London*, Discussion Papers in Economic and Social History, University of Oxford, p. 4.

Zaidel, D. W. 2014. Creativity, Brain, and Art: Biological and Neurological Considerations. *Frontiers in Human Neuroscience*, 8(June): 389.

6 Movement

KRIS SHARES A STORY

The Central Valley Suicide Hotline is housed in a nondescript strip mall which bears no sign. The other storefronts are empty and forlorn with dark windows shaded against the relentless sun. The howl of constant traffic fills the busy avenue, which is skirted by a broad sidewalk that rarely attracts pedestrians. As it is a recently constructed area, the planted trees are young and immature, giving little shade while pushing up against the beating sun. The hotline runs twenty-four hours a day, seven days a week, and employs a couple of social workers buttressed by a dozen volunteers, per diem workers, and a handful of student interns. A bevy of cars is parked next to the faceless entrance to the hotline center in the otherwise empty parking lot.

Suicide rates in the United States have risen dramatically in recent years, with the Centers for Disease Control and Prevention suggesting that there has been a 25% increase between 1999 and 2016 (Centers for Disease Control and Prevention, 2017). 'Deaths of despair' – meaning fatal drug overdoses, poisonings, accidents, alcoholic liver disease, and other acts of self-harm – are a growing epidemic. Nearly 50,000 Americans killed themselves in 2017 (Centers for Disease Control and Prevention, 2017). The population of white men in the United States, often considered the most categorically privileged group in the nation, are seeing a steep rise in self-inflicted fatalities (Metzl, 2020). According to Case and Deaton (2020, 40), deaths of despair among middle-aged white American rose from 31 to 91 per 100,000. Indigenous and Aboriginal communities globally have significantly higher rates of suicide than that of white populations in Australia, Canada, New Zealand, and the United States (Hatcher, 2016). Statistics Canada has estimated that the First Nations suicide rate is three times higher than the non-Indigenous population (Kumar and Tjepkema, 2019). The report emphasizes that that these high statistics do not necessarily represent the shortcomings of communities but demonstrate the complex legacy and historical trauma of settler colonialism.

As Émile Durkheim argued in the nineteenth century, suicide will rise unless people find a way to live meaningful and dignified lives. The collective weight of our deeply unequal and unhealthy twenty-first-century societies appears to undermining the ability to thrive (Case and Deaton, 2020). Social isolation, general anxiety, hopelessness, overwork, and acute psychological distress are pervasive throughout Western societies. In their study of self-destructive behavior in humans and our fellow creatures, medical historians Ramsden and Wilson (2014, 205) argue that "innate and unconscious responses to social and ecological pressures" is seen to be a driver of suicide.

At times, calling a hotline is the only opportunity a person has to connect with another person. Until 2013, the Central Valley had no community-based suicide prevention group, so when the hotline started, the lines lit up. Answering crisis calls is very stressful. Workers sit in small cubicles lit by florescent lights with no windows, typing on luminous computers. The phones ring constantly with complex calls that can involve alerting the authorities to rescue people or reporting child abuse. Sometimes the hotline workers have to spend time dealing with pranksters. Everything related to calls, including reports to the authorities, must be documented within a specific time frame, so workers sometimes have to stay later than their shift to finish paperwork. Dealing with never-ending crises, workers often run on adrenaline, chugging coffee and eating the doughnuts left in the break room to handle calls that can last for over two hours.

Current research estimates that office workers spend about 75% of their day sitting (Tobin, Leavy, and Jancey, 2016). Excessive sitting can cause a range of physical and psychological problems, from cardiovascular disease to increased risk of diabetes and depression. Considered one of the most important emerging public health risks, sedentary lifestyles are often hard to disrupt due to the way our workplaces have been constructed around technologies designed to keep our bodies stationary and focused on screens.

Dynamic, tough, and resourceful, dark-haired Azucena León is in her 30s and has three children. She is the supervising crisis social worker at the Central Valley Suicide Prevention Hotline and bears the heavy responsibility to ensure that calls are answered promptly and professionally by her ever-changing staff of workers and volunteers. Growing up in the impoverished San Joaquin Valley of California, she is devoted to her young local college interns who have faced many of the same struggles as Azucena. She closely guides, trains, and supports them to ensure their academic success, often writing them recommendations for graduate school. Many of her former interns have returned to work at the hotline as volunteers and even qualified social workers after graduation.

Azucena found that during the long shifts that she put in at the suicide prevention hotline, she rarely moved. Either engrossed in long conversations on the phone with distressed callers or sitting in working lunches, Azucena never stretched her legs or arms and spent long shifts inside without ever seeing the light of day. "My eyes were always looking at a computer screen," she said. "And I didn't feel good. I had constant headaches. I was tired all the time. I ended up getting thyroid cancer." Azucena had her thyroid partially removed and pushed through all of the treatments, yet she still didn't feel well. She was constantly fatigued and emotionally drained when she returned home. Azucena realized that her children were growing up quickly, and she did not want to miss out on spending time with them because she was too tired.

Azucena saw herself at a crossroads: She wanted to be at the hotline because the work is so important, especially in her underserved community with growing rates of suicide among youth. Yet sitting all day in front of a computer monitor did not leave her feeling well. Azucena asked herself whether she could do anything to change the situation. Azucena decided to try to find ways to move despite the limits of the work situation. Never able to stray far from the phone or desk, Azucena had to figure out how to move within these parameters. She started by bringing a workout shirt and tennis shoes every day to work. Looking up online videos on how to walk a mile in fifteen minutes, which was possible during her short break, Azucena would go outside around the building twice a day, walking quickly and punching the air. When others noticed what she was doing, they wanted to join in. Soon Azucena had many of the staff joining her, and they expanded their repertoire to indoor stretches and yoga. They laughed and joked with one another. She also began to bring healthier foods to the break room. A collective effort to be active and eat healthy brought a new sense of togetherness and sharing. There were no longer doughnuts in the break room; instead a variety of locally grown fruit and vegetables appeared. People started sharing recipes from their own cultures and families. Many of the workers started feeling more satisfied with their jobs and felt safer to reach out for support during the tough times.

Azucena's changes in her behavior and relationships are certainly better, and the office environment is happier and more supportive. But is this enough to keep her emotionally and physically healthy in the long run? Will walking fifteen minutes twice a day prevent Azucena from getting chronic diseases like obesity, diabetes, heart disease, dementia, and hypertension? While her gains are very positive, it may not fully counteract the deleterious conditions of her workplace. Our need for movement is more critical than ever, and more and more exercise research continues to conclude that those of us in Western industrial societies get far too little exercise. Social workers are increasingly laboring at jobs that promote ill-being rather than well-being. How can sedentary social workers who don't feel good promote well-being among clients? How can we social workers promote structural changes that transform the ways that we work and live to encourage healthy movement rather than expecting individuals to make incremental change?

Lessons on pathways

Our physical movement has been colonized by neoliberal notions of what it means to be productive in our personal and working lives in contemporary society. Repetitious occupational movements performed by meat processors, pipe fitters, and grocery store clerks cause specific injuries like carpal tunnel syndrome, bursitis, and tendonitis. Sitting for long periods in front of computers produces musculoskeletal strain and a higher risk for all causes of mortality (Diaz, Hutto, Howard et al., 2017). Neoliberal workplaces increasingly follow the movements and actions of workers through tracking devices and demands for precise, time-sensitive documentation, which control workers' bodies forcing them into repetitive movements or sedentary positions for long periods of time. The quantification of working life, especially through wearable devices that monitor all physical movements and even mood, is a new form of corporeal capitalism employed by huge corporations such as Amazon and Tesco that opens up terrifying new possibilities to control human behavior and undercuts the intrinsic right to be free in our own bodies (Moore and Robinson, 2016).

Our bodies are made to move and express themselves physically and emotionally in a variety of diverse ways. We experience, interpret, and feel the world through our physical bodies. Yet our colonizing systems have created a multitude of structural barriers to free physical mobility, which is increasingly becoming a privilege of the few. Children are shuttled back and forth by harried parents in cars, no longer able to walk safely and freely to school and recreational activities. Access to buildings, parks, and other amenities is often based on normative concepts of movement, presenting barriers to many. Workplaces control and monitor how and when we move. Opportunities to move have become ever more privatized as public spaces diminish because of enhanced loitering and trespass laws. Security fences and borders further inhibit free movement, presenting blockades for bodies bearing the wrong passport. And for many people of color or diverse genders, moving in the wrong area or in the wrong way can have lethal consequences.

The rise of the automobile in the twentieth century brought both mobility and restriction. Highways and motorways carved up the landscapes of many nations and can make walking and crossing streets dangerous. Pedestrian deaths are rising in many parts of the world, despite the fact that safety features in cars are better than ever (Baker, 2019). Freeways and suburbs often make it difficult to navigate cities in the United States and other places, in the sense that shopping and amenities are designed for cars instead of pedestrians. All of this development comes at a cost, with higher rates of poor physical fitness and increasing social distance from one another. Indeed, the rise of suburbia and reliance on the automobile has racially resegregated many American cities to a degree higher than the pre–Civil Rights era. The environmental consequences of suburbanization include vehicle dependence and increased air pollution, greater consumption of household fuel and other resources, and expanded land use with negative impacts on ecosystems (Kahn, 2000). But the sprawl of American suburbia, where each house has its own backyard and swimming pool, has begun to give way to urban gentrification along with the increasing privatization of public spaces. We have fewer public libraries and more Starbucks, less mass transit and more Google buses. All of these social changes have an impact on our ability to move among one another and even to know each other.

We live in societies that are constructed for normatively able-bodied people, societies which often actively create barriers to those with different abilities. Kris's apartment building in Helsinki, built in 1985, only has stairs, which makes it impossible for people with mobility issues to enter. The abundance of scooters zipping down the sidewalk and motorized robotic devices delivering food often creates a dangerous obstacle course for the aged, visually impaired, and people with mobility issues. We render invisible those with

different abilities and conceive of access points solely for those with normative abilities. Mobility equity thus requires thoughtful, adaptive, and universal
design so that movement does not become a privilege for those whose needs
are recognized and supported while shutting out others with different abilities
and requirements.

Movement is not just a matter of getting from one place to another; it is also a
means of creative expression and play. Play can be defined as activities that are
not purpose-driven and are engaged in for enjoyment, amusement, and relaxation.
We communicate through play and learn empathy by imagining being in the shoes
of others. Our emotions and sense of well-being in our bodies as well as our
minds. The neuroscience of play shows that both adults and children benefit in a
number of ways: Play increases one's positive emotional state, increases imagination and learning, stimulates creativity, and helps with socialization, bonding,
and exploration. Play is emblematic of both human and animal behavior. Lion
cubs roughhouse. Cats and coyotes pounce and engage in rough and tumble play
with companions. Dogs bow when they want to invite another canine to play.
Herring gulls play a group game of dropping and catching clam shells (Gamble
and Cristol, 2002). Human culture is imbued with play. In a 4,000-year old city in
Mohenjo-Daro in the Indus Valley, every tenth relic recovered through an archaeological dig was related to game playing (Graber, 2011). The Aztecs played a ball
game called *ullamaliztli*. The ancient Celts had a board game called *gwyddbwyll*
in Welsh or *fidhcheall* in Irish. Playing together through movement is a behavior
characteristic of all creatures.

To return to Azucena's story, we can see that she had to rediscover a sense
of play in movement to motivate herself as well as to mitigate the impact of the
limitations on her movement at work. Considering the deleterious health impact
of extended periods of sitting, it is worth asking how such important work could
be done differently. How can we move our bodies in ways that allow us to be free
and healthy? How can we rediscover the joy of moving and play? How can we
challenge the structures that keep us chained to our desks and sedentary or block
us due to our non-normative disabilities?

Decolonizing our relationship with movement

For tens of thousands of years, ancient peoples have observed and recorded the
movements of celestial bodies, animals, plants, weather patterns, and natural earth
and sea activity. Based upon these patterns, our ancestors created calendars, songs,
dances, ceremonies, and symbols to study and incorporate these movements into
their physical and spiritual being. For many cultural groups, movement is intimately connected to the sacred and the sexual, to health and social expressions.
We use our bodies in dance movements with diverse forms of physical, emotional, and spiritual expression. Northern Plains tribes in the United States had
dances that imitated the buffalo; the woodlands tribes and tribes in the southwest
had snake dances; tribes in southern California and Utah engaged in bear dances;
and tribes in Arizona and Mexico performed a deer dance. All of these types of

movements reflected a deep relationality with fellow creatures and Mother Earth and a sense of joy in collective play in movement.

Humans evolved to move. In traditional cultures, running, walking, dancing, hunting and gathering, planting, and harvesting are everyday ways of life. Through moving in relation with the natural world, Indigenous Peoples gained knowledge of botany, geology, fellow creatures, water, the stars, and many other aspects of Mother Earth. Indigenous ways of knowing do not separate the mind from the body, as Michi Saagiig Nishnaabeg scholar Leanne Betasamosake Simpson (2011, 42) notes, "In order to access knowledge from a Nishnaabeg perspective, we have to engage our entire bodies: our physical beings, emotional self, our spiritual energy and our intellect." Drawing from a holistic Indigenous methodology, Marin and Bang (2018) underline the growing use of ambulatory methods by social scientists to better understand people's relationship to place and spatial relationships. Richard M. Carpiano (2009), for example, developed the "go-along" qualitative method of understanding people's relationship to the health-related issues of neighborhoods and places. In this method, the researcher accompanies a participant on an outing in their neighborhood and, through asking questions and observing, learns more about the health context of the individual's relationship to place. By moving with participants rather than conducting sedentary interviews, Carpiano is able to convey his interest and respect to the community, experience the context, and reduce power differentials by empowering the participant to act as the leader (Carpiano, 2009, 267). Experiencing relationship to place and moving are deeply interconnected in decolonized approaches to knowing and being.

One of the joys of moving is not simply to get to the place one is headed efficiently but the freedom of meandering and being outside in nature and public space. Wordsworth's lyrical poem *I Wandered Lonely as a Cloud* foreshadows a fundamentally relational view of Mother Earth as the speaker experiences the pleasure of connection when happening upon daffodils in his wanderings. And as Rebecca Solnit points out in her history of walking, *Wanderlust* (2014, 10–11), the relentless focus of mobility technology has eradicated our chances to get lost in public spaces, depriving us not only of the time to daydream and woolgather but also of moving as a body in public with other bodies. To move nowadays, we often need to join a gym or buy a treadmill and even hire a coach to encourage us. Solnit further observes that the more that we are ensconced in private health clubs, automobiles, and gated communities, the more we lose connection with one another and the place where we are. The many technologies developed to improve our mobility (and the barriers that normalize access for certain bodies) have separated us from locomotion and community, which is an essential part of our being and relationality with others and place.

Decolonizing our relationship with movement starts by removing the artificial barrier that Western binary thinking has constructed between being, knowing, and moving-as-embodied acting. We have become alienated from our bodies through the internalization of the colonial gaze. Settler colonialists were imbued with Christian religions steeped in shame of the physical, particularly of the female body, and viewed bodies seen as non-white as 'savage,' 'animal-like,' and filled with wanton sexuality. Considering their own bodies as wicked and needing to be covered though the puritanical interpretations of Christianity instilled by the persecuting European society, settler colonialists projected sinfulness on to the bodies of Indigenous Peoples. Prevailing contemporary concepts of the right size, color, and shape of gendered bodies are rooted in colonized views of corporeality, or being in our body. In her book on the history of fat shame, Ann Farrell (2011) documents the links between moral outrage against fatness and emerging constructions of whiteness in industrial capitalism. Attitudes towards fatness reflect the complex relationship between excessive consumption, settler colonial Protestant concepts of self-denial, and racialized views of normalizing and judging the human body. Similarly, the medicalization of the differently abled body as deficit has informed ways that ability is evaluated and socially accepted. By inscribing shame on the bodies of racialized, gendered, and differently abled people, the ideology of settler colonialism has exerted control over how bodies encountered one another in the public realm. Fatphobia, ableism, sexism, homophobia, and transphobia are rooted in deep histories of oppressive colonizing frameworks that make us feel unsightly and unworthy of being and moving in public spaces.

Decolonizing movement starts with feeling comfortable, safe, and proud in our bodies and recognizing the intrinsic connection between mind, spirit, body, and place. This is difficult in oppressive colonial structures that continue to separate, erase, and judge us, making us ashamed of ourselves or frightened (often with good cause) to be in public spaces. In her book *Black Faces, White Spaces* (2014), Carolyn Finney discusses the complexity of the African American relationship to the environment within dominant narratives that delegitimize and pigeonhole people of color. The American city ordinances known as the "ugly laws" were mobilized to prohibit the disabled from being in public. In San Francisco of the 1970s, gay safe-streets patrols were started to mitigate the risks of being increasingly visible as out and proud (Hanhardt, 2008). Women and trans people have long curtailed their movement, knowing that being in the wrong place at the wrong time could lead to harm. Oppressive structures that define and shape place have a direct and powerful impact on our movement and sense of safety. Decolonizing movement means regenerating our fundamental connection with land and place through healing our bodies from the physical, social, and emotional violence of exclusion as well as feeling the intrinsic pleasure of being and moving in our bodies, but these changes can only come by decolonizing the structures that shape our lives and the places where we live.

Embodying our practice

Western science has been constructed on a binary that separates the body and the mind, privileging reason and the mind over the body, especially in medical and psychological healing. The body has often represented the intuitive and emotional and been associated with the feminine and viewed as inferior to the mind, which has been seen as rational and masculine. Conceptions of working as mental health professionals have been dominated by interventions that focus on the mind, from the deep psychoanalysis to cognitive-behavioral therapy. In popular representations of therapy from the American cartoonist Charles M. Schulz' cartoon character Lucy in *Peanuts* sitting in her booth to Sigmund Freud silently listening to his patients from his easy chair, the healing encounter is often constructed as a sedentary, mind-based, and largely unidirectional practice that separates the mind and body. The foundation of the social work curriculum continues to largely rest on psychodynamic and cognitive models of mental health despite increasing recognition of the important role that the moving body has in healing.

Consciousness in Western science has generally been constructed as neural and central nervous system activity, which is not constitutively dependent on the body (Maiese, 2010). There have been growing challenges to this dominant binary model in recent decades, grounded in theories like attachment and embodiment. Attachment theory was pioneered by John Bowlby, who studied separation and loss in children displaced by war or institutions. Bowlby's work underlined the importance of relational bonds and physical proximity between children and parents for healthy emotional and social development. Emerging from the philosophy of phenomenology, a school of thought called embodiment research would argue, in Linda Finlay's words, that "the body discloses the world just as the world discloses itself through the body" (2006, 19). The field of embodiment has emerged as a counterpoint to the exclusive focus on the mind. Cognitive embodiment "proposes that cognitive processes and knowledge itself are inseparable from our corporeal experience in the world" (Alessandroni, 2018, 228). In other words, our bodies process our minds and vice versa. Embodiment in social work encompasses many aspects of how social and biological factors such as poverty, stress, and trauma rest in our bodies and how acting through moving our bodies can be healing.

Tangenberg and Kemp (2002) argued for greater recognition of the complex relationship of the body in social work practice. Pointing out that social work practice is focused on the client in a myriad of embodied situations concerning abuse, trauma, grief, and other difficult matters, Tangenberg and Kemp note that because the body is such a given in social work, it is often taken for granted and ignored. The Western tradition of privileging the mind over the body also contributes to the 'disembodiment' of social work (Saleeby, 1992). Jeyasingham (2017) has explored how bodies move in social work through narratives by workers, observing that "social work bodies in these accounts were soft and malleable, able to morph into different shapes and sizes in order to get into places that are difficult to access." Thus, while social work is often seen as sedentary, it actually has many dynamic features of movement (in cars, across town, through institutional corridors, in family homes, and in relation to people). Social work practice is therefore never solely cognitive.

In their trailblazing book on integrative social work practice, *Integrative Body-Mind-Spirit Social Work*, Mo Yee Lee, Siu-man Ng, Pamela Pui Yu Leung, and Cecilia Lai Wan Chan (2009), speak of the limitations of verbal and mind-focused interventions that do not take into the many dimensions of human beings, including the corporeal and spiritual. Noting that neurocognitive research has demonstrated that memory is processed through the amygdala bypassing the cognitive part of the brain, these integrative social work practitioners emphasize the importance of expanding movement and kinesthetic awareness as key elements of healing "because clients need to use their bodies rather than just sitting, talking, or thinking, therapeutic sessions using body movement encourage the active participation and commitment of the client" (Lee at al., 2009, 168). Integrative social work practice recognizes that trauma exists in the disconnection of the mind from the body, and healing comes from their natural relationality. A recent study of recovering heroin users explored how they reported participating in and experiencing physical activity, such as cycling, playing sports, and other physical activity. Noting that "physical activity may be less about solving social problems and eradicating social inequalities than it is about enabling marginalized groups to relax, have fun and feel good for a while. Indeed, even routine activities of daily living, such as walking and cycling, can be an important source of pleasure and satisfaction," the researchers underline the intrinsic healing qualities of moving in our bodies (Neale, Nettleton, and Pickering, 2012, 126).

Increasingly, health care and social work practice has recognized the importance of movement and play in supporting well-being (Ergler, Kearns, and Witten, 2013). From healthy aging to child development programs, movement is becoming a growing focus of preventive physical and mental health (Daniels, Arena, Lavie, Cahalin, and Forman, 2013). Emerging notions of healthy aging have underlined the value of movement in supportive and accessible places in keeping bodies agile and minds active (Ivey, Kealey, Kurtovich, Hunter, Prohaska, Bayles, and Satariano, 2015). Play therapy has developed as a kinetic and imaginative means of working with the mental health needs of children (Swank, Shin, Cabrita, Cheung, and Rivers, 2015). Following attachment and cognitive embodiment theories, play has been seen as a means to decrease social isolation and enhance empathy and a sense of attachment and well-being (Maiese, Protevi, and Wheeler, 2010; Ryan and Edge, 2012; Wilson and Ray, 2018). Dance movement therapy has also integrated movement and play into social work practice (Murrock and Graor, 2016; Travaglia and Treefoot, 2010). Eye movement desensitization and reprocessing (EMDR) has promising treatment for trauma, tying physical movements to the psychic experience of trauma by retraining eye movements to better manage the physical cues of mental trauma (Leer, Engelhard, and van Den Hout, 2014). Traditional ceremonies of dance provide possibilities for people to heal (Weir, 2017). There are a great many other varieties of therapy and wellness activities that have emerged to bridge the mind-body divide.

The despair of disconnection so often reflected in suicide and addiction cannot always be managed solely through the mind. We wrote about the complexity of trauma in Chapter 2, pointing out that the heavy legacy of historical trauma does not fit into neat diagnostic boxes. Trauma is commonly recognized most clearly through physical symptoms, such as those displayed by shell shocked soldiers in the First World War who demonstrated compulsive movements, tics, and other physical disorders, or by the numbness and disconnection often displayed by survivors of sexual abuse. Embracing Indigenous ways of knowing could help open up the innate healing tie between mind and body by marshaling the power of movement in the body through communal ceremony, group dance, and individual exercise.

References

Alessandroni, N. 2018. Varieties of Embodiment in Cognitive Science. *Theory & Psychology*, 28(2): 227–248.

Baker, P. C. 2019. Collision Course: Why Are Cars Killing More and More Pedestrians? *The Guardian*. 3 October. Accessed 15 March 2020 at https://www.theguardian.com/technology/2019/oct/03/collision-course-pedestrian-deaths-rising-driverless-cars

Carpiano, R. M. 2009. Come Take a Walk with Me: The "Go-Along" Interview as a Novel Method for Studying the Implications of Place for Health and Well-being. *Health and Place*, 15(1): 263–272.

Case, A., and Deaton, A. 2020. *Deaths of Despair and the Future of Capitalism*. Princeton: Princeton University Press.

Centers for Disease Control and Prevention (CDC) Data & Statistics Fatal Injury Report for 2017.

Daniels, K., Arena, R., Lavie, C. J., Cahalin, L. P., and Forman, D. E. 2013. Exercise: A Vital Means to Moderate Cardiovascular Aging. *Aging Health*, 9(5): 473–482.

Diaz, K. M., Howard, V. J., Hutto, B., et al. 2017. Patterns of Sedentary Behavior and Mortality in US Middle-Aged and Older Adults: A National Cohort Study. *Annals of Internal Medicine*, 167: 465–475.

Ergler, C. R., Kearns, R. A., and Witten, K. 2013. Seasonal and Locational Variations in Children's Play: Implications for Wellbeing. *Social Science & Medicine*, 91: 178–185.

Farrell, A. 2011. *Fat Shame: Stigma and the Fat Body in American Culture*. New York: New York University Press.

Finlay, L. 2006. The Body's Disclosure in Phenomenological Research. *Qualitative Research in Psychology*, 3(1): 19–30.

Finney, C. 2014. *Black Faces, White Spaces: Reimagining the Relationship of African Americans to the Great Outdoors*. Chapel Hill: University of North Carolina Press.

Gamble, J. R., and Cristol, D. A. 2002. Drop-catch Behavior Is Play in Herring Gulls, Larus Argentatus. *Animal Behaviour*, 63(2): 339.

Graber, C. 2011. *Ancient People Played a Lot of Games*. Accessed 2 April 2018 at www.scientificamerican.com/podcast/episode/ancient-people-played-lots-of-games-11-02-09.

Hanhardt, C. 2008. Butterflies, Whistles, and Fists: Gay Safe Streets Patrols and the "New Gay Ghetto", 1976–1981. *Radical History Review*, 100: 61.

Hatcher, S. 2016. Indigenous Suicide: A Global Perspective with a New Zealand Focus. *The Canadian Journal of Psychiatry*, 61(11): 684–687.

Ivey, S. L., Kealey, M., Kurtovich, E., Hunter, R. H., Prohaska, T. R., Bayles, C. M., and Satariano, W. A. 2015. Neighborhood Characteristics and Depressive Symptoms in an Older Population. *Aging & Mental Health*, 19(8): 713–722.

Jeyasingham, D. 2017. Soft, Small, Malleable, and Slow: Corporeal Form and Movement in Social Workers' and Police Officers' Talk about Practice in a Multi-Agency Safeguarding Hub. *Child & Family Social Work*, 22: 1456–1463.

Kahn, M. 2000. The Environmental Impact of Suburbanization. *Journal of Policy Analysis and Management*, 19(4): 569–586.

Kumar, M., and Tjepkema, M. 2019. *National Household Survey: Suicide among First Nations people, Métis and Inuit (2011–2016): Findings from the 2011 Canadian Census Health and Environment Cohort (CanCHEC)*. Accessed at https://www150.statcan.gc.ca/n1/pub/99-011-x/99-011-x2019001-eng.htm.

Lee, M. Y., Ng, S.-M., Leung, P. P. Y., and Chan, C. 2009. *Integrative Body-Mind-Spirit Social Work: An Empirically Based Approach to Assessment and Treatment*. Oxford: Oxford University Press.

Leer, A., Engelhard, I., and van Den Hout, M. 2014. How Eye Movements in EMDR Work: Changes in Memory Vividness and Emotionality. *Journal of Behavior Therapy and Experimental Psychiatry*, 45(3): 396–401.

Maiese, M. 2010. *The Essential Embodiment Thesis. In: Embodiment, Emotion, and Cognition*. New Directions in Philosophy and Cognitive Science. Palgrave Macmillan, London.

Maiese, M., Protevi, J., and Wheeler, M. 2010. *Embodiment, Emotion, and Cognition*. Basingstoke: Palgrave Macmillan: [distributor] Not Avail.

Marin, A. S., and Bang, M. 2018. "Look It, This Is How You Know:" Family Forest Walks as a Context for Knowledge-Building About the Natural World. *Cognition and Instruction*, 36(2): 89–118.

Metzl, J. 2020. *Dying of Whiteness: How the Politics of Racial Resentment Is Killing America's Heartland*. S.l.: Basic Books.

Moore, P., and Robinson, A. 2016. The Quantified Self: What Counts in the Neoliberal Workplace. *New Media & Society*, 18(11): 2774–2792.

Murrock, C. J., and Graor, C. H. 2016. Depression, Social Isolation, and the Lived Experience of Dancing in Disadvantaged Adults. *Archives of Psychiatric Nursing*, 30(1): 27–34.

Neale, J., Nettleton, S., and Pickering, L. 2012. Heroin Users' Views and Experiences of Physical Activity, Sport and Exercise. *International Journal of Drug Policy*, 23(2): 120–127.

Ramsden, E., and Wilson, D. 2014. The Suicidal Animal: Science and the Nature of Self-Destruction. *Past & Present*, 224(1): 201–242.

Ryan, V., and Edge, A. 2012. The Role of Play Themes in Non-directive Play Therapy. *Clinical Child Psychology and Psychiatry*, 17(3): 354–369.

Saleebey, D. 1992. Biology's Challenge to Social Work: Embodying the Person-in-Environment Perspective. *Social Work*, 37(2): 112–118.

Simpson, L. 2011. *Dancing on Our Turtle's Back: Stories of Nishnaabeg Re-creation, Resurgence and a New Emergence*. Winnipeg, Canada: Arbeiter Ring.

Solnit, R. 2014. *Wanderlust: A History of Walking*. London: Granta.

Swank, J., Shin, S., Cabrita, C., Cheung, C., and Rivers, B. 2015. Initial Investigation of Nature-Based, Child-Centered Play Therapy: A Single-Case Design. *Journal of Counseling and Development*, 93(4): 440–450.

Tangenberg, K. M., and Kemp, S. 2002. Embodied Practice: Claiming the Body's Experience, Agency, and Knowledge for Social Work. *Social Work*, 47(1): 9–18.

Tobin, R., Leavy, J., and Jancey, J. 2016. Uprising: An Examination of Sit-stand Workstations, Mental Health and Work Ability in Sedentary Office Workers, in Western Australia. *Work (Reading, Mass.)*, 55(2): 359.

Travaglia, R., and Treefoot, A. 2010. Exploring the Dance and Music Dialogue: Collaboration Between Music Therapy and Dance Movement Therapy in Aotearoa/New Zealand. *The New Zealand Journal of Music Therapy*, 8: 34–58.

Weir, A. 2017. Collective Love as Public Freedom: Dancing Resistance. Ehrenreich, Arendt, Kristeva, and Idle No More. *Hypatia*, 32(1): 19–34.

Wilson, B. J., and Ray, D. 2018. Child-Centered Play Therapy: Aggression, Empathy, and Self-Regulation. *Journal of Counseling & Development*, 96(4): 399–409.

7 Quiet and contemplation

KRIS SHARES A STORY

Seeking to spin Finland's reputation for ponderous quiet as a positive alternative to the cluttered, hectic, and frazzled rush of contemporary life, the Finnish Tourist Board in 2011 initiated a marketing campaign that called for "Silence, please." With lush photographs of green rural landscapes and simple interior designs largely devoid of people, the Visit Finland website promised a calm, clean, and simple way of life for visitors that could even provide healing.

As a peripheral country in the northwestern corner of the European Union between Russia and Sweden, Finland was long seen as a rather provincial nation famous mainly for its ski jumpers and reindeer. Owing to an inscrutable language and long, dark winters, Finnish society and culture remained largely unknown to outsiders. A famous aversion to small talk and casual conversation props up the stereotype of silent Finns, reinforced recently with online memes of tightlipped Formula One driver Kimi Räikkönen and Finnish people standing at a good distance from one another at bus stops. Reflecting on the bilingual nation, Bertolt Brecht once said that Finns can be "silent in two languages." And a frequently told joke goes as that two Finns are traveling by ferry to Sweden, they sit at the bar and drink. After a few hours, one says to the other: "This is good vodka, no?" The other responds after a long pause: "Did you come here to talk or drink?" Notions of Finnish silence and awkwardness in social situations are legendary. The challenge for the Finnish Tourist Board was how to cultivate this curious reputation and market it to construct Finland as a desirable destination.

Advantageously for Finland, tourists have increasingly sought to find places away from the beaten track that offer a variety of experiences. Since the success of Elizabeth Gilbert's book *Eat, Pray, Love*, for example, thousands of spiritual tourists have descended upon Bali seeking balance and inner peace. As spiritual tourism numbers leap, there has been increasing discussion about the ethics its impact on local economics and religious sites in terms of sustainable development. Spas, yoga retreats, and ecotourism have all become major trends in the travel industry, but spiritual tourism has a long history. *The International Journal of Religious Tourism and Pilgrimage* is devoted to exploring all aspects of spiritual journeys. For centuries, spiritual tourists have journeyed to sacred places in search of enlightenment, often through the practice of the pilgrimage. Seeking to become closer to the divine or to make penance for wrongs, pilgrims embark on a difficult or rigorous peregrination in search of spiritual awakening: People have climbed the arduous Kumano Kodo in Japan for over a thousand years, intending to worship at sacred Shinto shrines and Buddhist temples. And Croagh Patrick in County Mayo, Ireland, is a steep summit which many climb barefoot to perform penance, though it may have pre-Christian origins. In Islam, shrines create a spiritual landscape which culminate in the Hajj in Mecca, attracting up to two million pilgrims annually. Religious pilgrimages are often tied to venerating relics and places. Pilgrimage may be associated with a religion, but the concept is often borrowed for more existential spiritual quests for meaning in a complex and confusing world where the point is the difficulty of the journey.

Silence is often used in prayer, retreats, and pilgrimages as a means to connect with the divine essence of the universe. Seen as a powerful tool to quiet the restless mind and focus attention, silence is also a critical practice. Activists have long used silence and long marches as a means to draw attention to social injustice. In 1917, the Negro Silent Protest Parade was organized in New York City to demonstrate against lynchings in the aftermath of riots in East St. Louis. In 1930, thousands followed Mohandas Gandhi from his religious retreat to the sea on the famous Salt March to protest a British tax. Colin Kaepernick, an American football player, held regular silent kneeling protests at the playing of the national anthem at the beginning of games. Silent protest has been used as a form of public ritual to witness and acknowledge injustice and to hold space for victims or survivors. The transformative practice of silence "in public life resists single interpretations and opens up possibilities for new understandings of the political" (Hatzisavvidou, 2015, 511). Silence thus both resists and elicits interpretation (Ferguson, 2003).

Along with contemporary spiritual quests for awakening and protest against the structures of society, there has been a growing emphasis on quiet and slowness in contrast to the velocity of modern life. The slow living movement started with slow food (in contrast to fast food) at the beginning of the 1990s, reflecting the aim to be sustainable, local, organic, and whole (Parkins and Craig, 2006). Notions of slow have been connected with the absence of noise and distraction and focus on the task at hand. This has also given rise to the popularity of silent retreats, in which participants often pay high prices to hand over electronic devices and sit in silence with strangers for days or even weeks. Many have reported that the experience has led to less anxiety, clarity about priorities, and a greater sense of equanimity and peacefulness (Pagis, 2015).

By presenting the country as a place where it is possible to breathe and be quiet in the midst of a busy urban landscape, the Visit Finland campaign targeted the exhaustion many feel living in the seething world of social media, canned music, and traffic. The ability to turn off and be silent are increasingly becoming a luxury available only to the few. Hence, the Finnish marketing campaign strikes a deep chord with tourists who will pay to be left alone.

Lessons on pathways

Technology has brought us closer together than even and also isolated us more than ever. Some talk about the 'lizard brain,' referring to the limbic cortex, which controls our most primitive instincts, such as fight or flight, as being activated by the dopamine hits of 'persuasive technology' to influence our behavior (Parkin, 2018). We are constantly surrounded by the technological clutter that begs for our attention – Facebook notifications, text messages, tight deadlines, and the glow of screens – and make us hypervigilant and often anxious. Our brains are constantly engaged in tidal wave of messages that chronically mobilize our stress response at the expense of our physical and mental health.

We live in a maelstrom of noise: cars honk, telephones trill, televisions yak in waiting rooms, jackhammers drill, leaf blowers roar in our neighborhoods. We eat in restaurants where we have to shout to be heard by our companions. We wear ear protectors to enjoy the music at the rock concerts we attend. We sit at stoplights in cars with speakers bumping beats that make our windows vibrate. An exploratory study in New York City found high levels of street noise even in urban parks, which placed over 90% of study participants over the Environmental Protection Agency's recommended 70-decibel exposure limit (McAlexander, Gershon, and Neitzel, 2015). We seek to escape the constant hullabaloo by wearing earphones, although that places us at greater risk of death and injury in our environments, where we could be hit by cars or mugged (Williams, 2005).

The noise we abhor, even if only subconsciously, causes psychosocial and physiological effects in the form of sleep disturbance, anxiety, annoyance, and cardiovascular and other health issues (Goines and Hagler, 2007). Studies have shown that excessive noise has an impact on stress levels, hearing loss, and autonomic nerve function, causing high blood pressure and heart arrythmia, as well as sleep disturbance and even lost productivity (Botteldooren, 2011). One study showed an association between self-reported exposure to noise and infant congenital anomalies (Zhang, Cai, and Lee, 1992). Over 20 million residents of the United States have non-work-related hearing loss, with 40 million US adults experiencing significant hearing loss (Voelker, 2017). Noise is a public health crisis.

Cognizant of the hazards of noise, countries around the world have passed noise abatement laws to protect people from intrusive sound from airports, concerts, and construction sites, among other activities. Defined as "unwanted or disturbing sound" by the US Environmental Protection Agency, noise has been recognized by public health authorities since the 1960s as a health risk. In recognition of the dangers of noise pollution, the Noise Pollution and Abatement Act became law in 1972 in the United States. This law linked land use proposals with noise abatement targeting areas such as airports, construction sites, and transportation routes. However, it was defunded by the federal government in 1981, leaving state and local governments to manage noise pollution.

Law enforcement interventions often define noise by dominant communities seeking to smother the sound-making activities of marginalized peoples. In her study of street noise in Harlem, Clare Corbould (2007, 859) notes that the cacophony of sound represented a "multiplicity of voices [that] was ultimately the defining characteristic of the Black public sphere." This soundscape of identity and inclusion was heard as noise by outsiders. Sound and vibration, as we with music, play an important role in transmitting energy between matter as well as enhancing communication. Hence, what is considered bothersome noise depends on the context and the power relations surrounding the sound.

Noise has increased as populations around the world have exploded and become urbanized. Consumer lifestyles use greater resources swallowing up open space through sprawl, proliferating highways, deforestation, and other land management interventions. Even when we go to national parks in search of peace and quiet, humans bring noise that alters the soundscape to the detriment of animals and wildlife. Indeed, studies have shown that human noise affects animal behavior, including how they search for food, which has serious implications for preservation of natural habitats and endangered species. It is hard to deny that our globe has spun into a ball of confusion.

The term *noise* is not just sonic but also describes unwanted disturbance or irrelevant data. As technology keeps us constantly connected through social media and the internet, we find ourselves in a state of perpetual awareness and reactivity that fundamentally alters our brain function, interfering with our capacity to focus and concentrate. Our work culture demands that we are always on and at the ready with our devices. Our social life revolves around sharing photos of the food we have eaten and continually checking the status of our friends. We feel fidgety without our devices and are constantly seeking the dopamine rush of instant access to information. As one technology journalist puts it, "What the Net seems to be doing is chipping away my capacity for concentration and contemplation. Whether I'm online or not, my mind now expects to take information the way the Net distributes it: in a swiftly moving stream of particles. Once I was a scuba diver in the sea of words. Now I zip along the surface on a jet ski" (Carr, 2010, 47).

The opposite of, or antidote to, surface thinking could be mindfulness, which in contemporary, Western contexts takes many forms. One of the most popular definitions comes from Jon Kabat-Zinn, who calls mindfulness "the awareness that arises from paying attention, on purpose, in the present moment and non-judgmentally" (Kabat-Zinn, in Purser, 2015). In his second edition of his book, *Full Catastrophe Living*, Kabat-Zinn (2013) now says,

> Over the years, I have increasingly come to realize that mindfulness is essentially about relationality – in other words, *how we are in a relationship to everything*.
>
> (*p. xxxviii*)

However, many, but not all, in the Western-based movement have missed this second definition promoted by Kabat-Zinn and used mindfulness to cope individually with social injustice, climate change, racism, and colonization. Mindfulness has been largely promoted as a panacea to many of our contemporary social and medical ailments rather than our personal and collective responsibility toward one another and our Mother Earth.

In rather obscene fashion, many corporations, including those that engage in profits over people and environment, boast that the inclusion of mindfulness practices in their organizations enhances productivity, reduces workplace conflict and stress, and prevents burnout, which, of course, is all in the best interests of employee well-being – and profits. The premise of corporate mindfulness is that employees can manage their anxiety and minds and even increase their happiness through meditation techniques because stress is self-imposed through a lack of emotional self-regulation (Purser, Ng, and Walsh, 2017) and has nothing to do with the demands and unethical choices that these organizations leave their employees with: for instance, pressures to maintain company harmony but not reporting acts of racism and sexual harassment or putting up with token maternity leave for mothers for fear of losing their jobs. To this end, organizational behaviorist Jeffrey Pfeiffer (2018) indicates that workplace stress is largely due to the management practices of long hours, job insecurity, and the lack of work-life balance rather than a lack of stress management. Mindfulness cannot change the structural oppression of capitalism when the means are superficial, and the ends are profit over justice and ethics.

Corporate mindfulness reflects a bankrupt spiritual colonialism in its casual appropriation of complex and ancient practices that are were created for and embedded in a deeper sense of interconnectedness with others and nature. Some of the best representations of this relationship come from Indigenous Peoples around the world. In Aotearoa (New Zealand), Indigenous Māori communities still perform the Powhiri, a traditional ceremony to welcome guests with traditional songs, speeches, and foods, which signify a connection with others. The Yanomami of the Brazilian rainforest, a hunter-gatherer group, maintains high regard for sharing and equality, and the hunters among the tribe will not eat an animal that they have killed but instead distribute it equally among all tribal members. In Australia, the corroboree dancing ceremony of Aboriginal peoples is associated with culture, land, community, dreamtime, and beliefs. Many North American Indigenous tribes continue to practice ceremonies that pay respect for earth, lands, and animals. The Muckleshoot, who live on the coast the Puget Sound in Washington State, still practice the First Salmon Ceremony, in which the entire community shares the first caught Spring Chinook. Following the feast, the remains of the fish are put back in the river where it was caught so that its spirit can tell other salmon how well it was taken care of. In the Great Plains of the United States and Canada and throughout North America, many diverse Indigenous tribes gather to acknowledge all life, build a healing community, and pray for the well-being of all people and the planet through their participation in the Sun Dance ceremony that occurs during the summer months.

In what follows, we critically consider how quiet and contemplation has been an integral part of most traditional Indigenous cultures and what this implies for healing. We ponder the role of quiet in the noisy world of social work practice. In this chapter, we ask: How can slowing down, acting deliberately, cultivating quiet, deeply connecting, and drawing on an authentic decolonized mindfulness heal us as social workers – and our clients?

Decolonizing noise

In the Western scientific creation story, the universe emerged from a big bang. Contemporary physics and mystic traditions hold that everything in the universe vibrates at different speeds and frequencies, which means that all reality is essentially sound. Sounds travels in waves and requires a medium, such as objects, gases, or liquids, to vibrate and move. Similar to the story of the Big Bang, many Indigenous Peoples have creation myths that begin with sound. The Laguna Pueblo people believe that the world was sung into existence by a woman:

> In the center of the universe she sang. In the midst of the waters she sang. In the midst of heaven she sang. In the center she sang. Her singing made all the worlds. The worlds of the Spirits. The worlds of the people. The worlds of the creatures. The worlds of the gods. In this way she separated the quarters. Singing, she separated. Upon the face of heaven she placed her song. Upon the face of water she placed her song. Thus she placed her song.
>
> (Harvey, 2005, 33)

All the universe vibrates, and we are always enclosed in some kind of sound. But what makes the difference between sound and noise? Is quiet the same as silence? Many community battles have been waged over our common soundscape, with advocates for or against disturbing noise. How can we decolonize quiet without enforcing class, race, and gendered notions of noise abatement? Can we have mindful contemplation with sound and ceremony? A quiet and authentic decolonized mindfulness could look any number of ways.

Settler colonialism brought what Diane Collins (2006) has called the "acoustics of exploration." Explorers coming from rapidly industrializing urban centers brought a new sonic experience to the lands that they invaded, and through sound, they sought to enforce order. The mechanized noise of the city and industry, for example, contrasted with that of the 'wild' (Collins, 2006, 3). The shriek of the factory whistle marking the beginning and ending times of work and the roar of the factories manufacturing goods from resources transported on thundering trains produced a new auditory world of settler colonialism (Collins, 2006). Romantic notions of the countryside often hark to church bells and cows lowing, which can be seen as symbols of mans' domination of nature (and we mean man deliberately). The acoustics of Indigenous territories were profoundly unsettling to settler colonizers because they did not reflect the acoustics of domination. The wide-open spaces of Indigenous lands were not silent places but filled with sound, such as bison moving, birds migrating, and coyotes howling (Hurley, 2019). Quiet in 'the wild' was experienced in a profoundly different way than quiet in 'the countryside.' Quiet is therefore not the absence of all sound but is the lack of what is defined as noise.

What colonizers viewed as silence was often used as a reason to conquer because it was it equated with nothingness. Affirming and establishing sound became one element of the settler colonial ordering of the world and a means of asserting domination (Collins, 2006, 16). Indigenous lands were unsettling precisely because they did not play the soundtrack of industrial capitalism. The wild or quietness did not sound how an empire should sound. To decolonize noise, our understanding of quiet must be reconfigured, and we must return to being comfortable with the sounds of a noncolonial world.

Ancient and Indigenous cultures around the world have contemplative traditions that have served to heal people through connection to the past. There are deep traditions throughout the world of altered states of consciousness through deep contemplation. Shamanism, for example, is one of the oldest spiritual practices of human beings with the term originating with the Evenki people in trans Russia-China (Heyne, 2000). A key element of shamanism is the recognition that there is the world that is seen and that which is not, though both worlds are deeply intertwined. Among Aboriginal peoples in Australia, this is called 'dreamtime,' while ancient Celts called it 'the other world,' and many Indigenous cultures referred to the 'spirit world.' Shamanic experiences start with focused contemplation that leads to 'soul flight,' which means traveling from the known world to the unseen world. These travels are considered ways of healing and reaching deeper understanding. These acts of contemplation are sometimes silent, but more often not. In the Hmong tradition, 'soul calling' is a ritual in which a shaman goes into a trance to visit spirits on the other side to help guide the soul back into the body of the person under care. When this ceremony takes place, people often move around and visit.

Moving away from noise and into contemplative stillness requires a decolonization of the mind. A colonized mind revolves around the busyness and noise of the everyday. A colonized mind focuses on continuous production and requires a split from the holism of relationality and connection towards fragmentation and disconnection. The first step towards freedom from inner colonization thus comes from decolonizing ways of being. Quiet and contemplation allows for connection to all of creation around us, mental spaciousness, and deep awareness of the present moment.

The next step towards freedom from inner colonization comes from decolonizing ways of knowing, thinking, and speaking. Colonization enforces the uses the words, sounds, and concepts of the oppressor. African novelist Ngũgĩ wa Thiong'o (2011) wrote that imperialism is palpable in the very words used by colonized peoples through the loss of the diversity of native tongues. Writing about his childhood, wa Thiong'o recalled how the stories of fellow creatures and relatives all melded together through the lesson of mutual cooperation as the means of benefitting all in the community through his native language of Kikuyu. Decolonizing the mind starts from recognizing that the loss of one's own sounds through the imposition of an oppressor's language and sound making erases our connection with our heritage. By acting to revitalize our native tongues, sounds, and noise, we embrace our being and our relationality with our ancestors, fellow creatures, and the land.

Another step towards freedom from inner colonization comes from decolonizing ways of acting. Kimine Mayuzumi (2006) explored the meaning of the Japanese tea ceremony as mindful action. Initially thinking that the Japanese tea ceremony was rigid and even sexist because each bodily movement by the women serving the tea is so closely defined, such as how chopsticks or tea cup are held, Mayuzumi began to see how the ceremony actually connected mind, body, and the material world through decolonizing action in a healing way. Drawing from Indigenous ways of knowing, Mayuzumi notes how the tea ceremony connects the tea server to her roots with the ancestors by following closely prescribed actions that have been practiced for hundreds of years. The proverb *Ichigo ichie* (one encounter at a time) is used, according to Mayuzumi, to focus attention on the significance of each unique moment. The ceremony slows down time and creates focus. It is an exercise in contemplative ritual, connecting the present with the ancestors.

Neurodecolonization as healing

Successful decolonization first begins in the mind. The Buddha once said, "The mind is everything. What you think you become." Examining a preponderance of neuroscience research, Sharon Begley (2007) concludes that when one trains their mind, they change their brain and develop extraordinary potential for transformation. In this section, we introduce a decolonization approach called neurodecolonization, which is concerned with how the human mind and brain operate in a colonial context and how mindful decolonization[1] practices can enable a person and a community to purify, restructure, and decolonize the mind to overcome and transform colonial trauma, distractions, symbols, language, and systemic racism, sexism, ableism, and homophobia. The brain is the physical organ that changes its structure and function according to the needs of our mind, and the mind might be thought of as our perceptions, higher-order thinking, and consciousness. (Yellow Bird, 2013). The concept of neurodecolonization is informed and guided by concept of "neuroplasticity," which refers to our brain's capacity to change its structure and to accommodate new learning and experiences. Far from being an immutable physical structure, the brain has the capacity to remodel and adapt to new situations with neural networks becoming denser and functioning dynamically throughout our lives. (Demarin, Morović, and Béné, 2014).

There has long been a binary between biological and social science explanatory frameworks of human behavior. Until recently, modern biological science generally held that the mammalian brain was like a complex machine with fixed, unchanging parts. Epigenetics, the study of how gene activity and expression changes through outside influences, emerged in the late twentieth century, challenging dominant views of the unchanging brain. Epigenetics demonstrated the neuroplasticity of the brain, showing that cognitive behavioral therapy and mindfulness training could not only change thought patterns, for example, by lessening anxiety and depression but also alter neurological patterns of brain function assessed through MRI testing (Jokić-Begić, 2010; Kandel, 2006). Social science theories have increasingly recognized neuroplasticity as an important aspect of human development throughout the lifespan (Simons and Klopack, 2015). Recent research further indicates that oppressive phenomena, such as historical trauma, are transferred biologically through pathways in the brain to produce epigenetic change, resulting in poorer psychological and health outcomes down through the generations in complex ways (Conching and Thayer, 2019).

The aim of mindful neurodecolonization is training the mind to challenge destructive thoughts, feelings, emotions, and behaviors, especially those associated with historical trauma and contemporary oppression, which will enable the brain to make the necessary functional and structural changes to engage in these challenges (Yellow Bird, 2013). Neurodecolonization is a set of mindful decolonization practices that seek to restore balance, harmony, and resilience to the mind to promote healthy behaviors and thoughts while courageously and intelligently transforming structural oppression. Because colonialism thrives on control and domination, it promotes negative self-esteem, despair, and self-doubt, oppressive structures and ideologies, and destructive emotions. Colonialism beats down and bullies individuals and communities that oppose and resist destructive settler structures, ideologies, and processes. Bullying works, and there is substantial evidence that bullying, abuse, and negative stereotypes adversely impact our brain function, creating chronic stress, affecting our physical health, and causing intergenerational trauma (Meloni, Müller, and Manusy, 2018; Pedersen, Nuetzman, Gubbels, and Hummel, 2018). Decolonizing mindful practices are intended to challenge colonialism and create opportunities for community transformation and growth by privileging and engaging in Indigenous philosophies and practices that stabilize and build the cognitive resilience needed to counter colonialism and restore well-being. By using the mind to strip away the harmful and invasive beliefs of colonialism, the brain can begin the important task of restoring dignity, courage, and a warrior mindset that is capable of fully embracing and appreciating oneself to become empowered in new ways of being and acting in the world.

Overcoming colonialism is not a spectator sport that only Indigenous Peoples are responsible for. Decolonizing the minds of settlers is critical if there is going to be any reasonable chance to bring about the collapse of colonialism. Neurodecolonization is intended to bring settler allies into the colonialism war to openly support and build allyship with Indigenous Peoples. Neurodecolonization invites settlers to engage with Indigenous Peoples in mindful decolonization practices that are transformative and enable the growth of creative and healthy decolonized ways of being, thinking, and connecting in relationship with others to challenge the limitations and stressors of colonized thinking. Colonialism has created despair, confusion, and negative thinking in both settlers and Indigenous Peoples. It has taken an enormous toll on our physical bodies as well as emotions, often paralyzing us from seeing our situations clearly due to fear, anger, and hopelessness. Mindful decolonization is an act of healing, an act of resistance and a revolution of the mind, brain, and spirit intended to extinguish the anguish of living in colonial structures with the belief that colonialism is too big, too abstract, or too difficult to be overcome and transformed.

The practice of mindful decolonization can be done in many different ways. Below is one a mindful decolonization exercise you can practice and discuss with others. We invite you to join in this exercise as a way to explore your own thoughts and feelings about decolonizing your mind and the continuing effects of colonization on ourselves and our societies:

Activity

A mindful decolonization exercise: decolonizing the mind, decolonizing relationships, taking action

This exercise is best done by being in the natural setting. If this is not possible, you can do a sitting practice and imagine being in this place and taking action. While this practice is done with the forest setting, you can adapt it to any situation or place.

> Begin by sitting quietly on the floor or in a chair. Make sure you keep your back straight but relaxed and your neck aligned with your spine. Close your eyes if you like, or you can keep them slightly open as you focus on an area in front of you or on the floor. If you are sitting in a chair, make sure that both feet are resting on the floor. Relax your shoulders and put your hands, palms down, on the top of your legs. If you are sitting on the floor, rest your hands on your lap. One hand can rest inside the other, with your palms facing upward, fingers slightly and gently curled up, and thumbs lightly touching.
>
> When you are ready, begin breathing in and out, focusing on each breath as you gently allow each breath to enter your nostrils, descend down your windpipe, enter your lungs, and fill your entire body. Your breathing should be natural, even, and calm. As you breathe out, focus on your breath leaving your body, traveling up and exiting your nose. Continue this relaxed, even, mindful breathing for a minute or two.
>
> Imagine with each in-breath, you are inviting into your mind and body a strong sense of resilience, optimism, and calm. With each out-breath, you are seeing yourself releasing negative emotions, self-doubt, and reactivity. Continue this for a few minutes. If at any point you become distracted and lose the point of the exercise, simply come back to your breathing and begin again without judgement or frustration. Decolonizing the breath comes with practice.

Now imagine you are walking through a forest, smelling the fragrances of the flowers and plants, feeling the earth beneath you, and you are seeing the beauty and sounds or quiet of nature. Next, you can visualize seeing yourself as an integral part of the forest breathing and exchanging your breath with that of trees, plants, insects, and animals, understanding that they have an important role and stake in the ownership of the forest. As you train your mind to open up to the unjust political realities of colonialism, you now know that you must acknowledge that the forest you are in belonged to Indigenous Peoples and was stolen away from them by the city you live in and it must be returned or reparations must be made.

Perhaps you can feel the anguish they felt losing their forest and the consequences it had for their well-being. As you train your mind for just outcomes, you can now see yourself and others working to return this space to the rightful owners. You can practice seeing yourself engaging in actions to accomplish this: maybe speaking up to other settlers on behalf of Indigenous Peoples who live and own this forest; formally educating others about the colonization of this forest and the need to repatriate back it back to the owners. If you or others you know own land or property in this forest, you can train your mind to see yourself and others giving it back to Indigenous Peoples or making space to share it with them. When you are done with your meditation you can talk others and begin practicing your potential to decolonize the attitudes and ownership of this forest and help return it to the rightful owners.

As you do you do this mindful decolonization exercise, make sure you push yourself just a bit each time to understand that your mind is going through an important process of decolonization and that there is a purpose in what you are doing. Mindful decolonization is a radical, loving act that has the capacity to change you and your allies and transform the world around you for the highest good.

At some point, you can do this practice in a group. When you finish, you can discuss how you felt after practicing this exercise. Listen mindfully to one another without interruption or attempting to analyze someone's experiences when they share. Just listen. Were some parts of the exercise easier or more difficult? How so? Did your mind or breath feel colonized as if what you were doing was too difficult, stressful or ridiculous? Did it feel like it has been invaded and manipulated by outside forces and that it belongs to distractions, emotions, or content rather that you? Did the practice make you question the value of what you were doing and create self-doubt, or did it validate your beliefs? How do you think it relates to your understanding of neurodecolonization? What can you do to make it a more powerful, meaningful exercise that will lead to individual and community healing, structural change, and justice?

As we have discussed in previous chapters, colonization was born of a subjectivity that radically altered humans' traditional relationship to the natural world, themselves, and one another. Though conflict and aggressive behavior have been attributes of human beings from time immemorial, evolutionary survival required groups of people to altruistically cooperate and collaborate to maximize a balanced use of limited resources and provide security for all. However, during the period of European colonization, obsessive concern with resource extraction and profit combined with accelerating technology and increasingly impersonal systems of domination to create inequitable societies: materially wealthy, psychologically damaged, and now in imminent danger of extinction.

In the midst of climate crisis and the potential sixth extinction, we find ourselves surrounded by noise, unable to focus, filled with anxiety, and in ill health. Epigenetics points to the fact that postcolonial trauma continues to resonate down through the generations at the high personal and community cost of poor physical and mental health. The profession of social work is specifically tasked with working to empower and liberate oppressed and distressed individuals and groups.

Yet contemporary ways of conceiving of social work limit our ways of thinking and understanding our contemporary society and ways of healing because of the field's professionalization, a limited epistemology narrowly focusing on what constitutes "evidence-based outcomes," and personal change without challenging colonizing structures of oppression. This type of social work does not produce healing or true empowerment but rather dependence on the system of care and control.

Neurodecolonization is the contemplative science of healing that starts from quietening the mind to restore balance. It is based on the principle that to gain collective healing, we must start with ourselves by training our brains to promote resiliency. This process requires accountability and self-governance, recognizing the deep role of institutions and oppressive structures in our psyches. We have learned to adapt to colonized society for so long that we no longer have cognitive flexibility because we are bonded to noise, damaged beliefs, and our suffering. Decolonizing the mind means realizing its capacity to change – to throw off the chains of colonial limitations. It is futile to avoid difficult thoughts, but through neurodecolonization and relationality, individuals can build powerful healing tools to realize that their ancestors are with them. Neurodecolonization helps ready them for transformation.

Note

1 In this section, I use the terms *neurodecolonization* and *mindful decolonization* interchangeably.

References

Begley, S. 2007. *Change Your Mind, Change Your Brain: How a New Science Reveals Our Extraordinary Potential to Transform Ourselves*. New York: Ballantine Books.

Botteldooren, D. 2011. Measuring Noise for Health Impact Assessment. In *Encyclopedia of Environmental Health*, edited by Jerome O Nriagu, 3: 646–654. London: Elsevier Science.

Carr, N. 2010. *The Shallows: How the Internet Is Changing the Way We Think, Read and Remember*. New York: WW Norton.

Conching, A. K. S., and Thayer, Z. 2019. Biological Pathways for Historical Trauma to Affect Health: A Conceptual Model Focusing on Epigenetic Modifications. *Social Science & Medicine*, 230: 74–82.

Corbould, C. 2007. Streets, Sounds and Identity in Interwar Harlem. *Journal of Social History*, 40(4): 859–894.

Demarin, V., Morović, S., and Béné, R. 2014. Neuroplasticity. *Periodicum Biologorum*, 116(2): 209–211.

Diane, C. 2006. Acoustic Journeys: Exploration and the Search for an Aural History of Australia. *Australian Historical Studies*, 37(128): 1–17.

Ferguson, K. 2003. Silence: A Politics. *Contemporary Political Theory*, 2(1): 49.

Goines, L., and Hagler, L. 2007. Noise Pollution: A Modern Plague. *Southern Medical Journal*, 100(3): 287–294.

Harvey, G. 2005. *Animism: Respecting the Living World*. London: Hurst & Co.

Hatzisavvidou, S. 2015. Disturbing Binaries in Political Thought: Silence as Political Activism. *Social Movement Studies*, 14(5): 509–522,

Heyne, F. G. 2000. The Social Significance of the Shaman Among the Chinese Reindeer-Evenki. *Asian Folklore Studies*, 58(2): 377.

Hurley, A. W. 2019. Whistling the Death March? Listening in to the Acoustics of Ludwig Leichhardt's Australian Exploration. *Australian Historical Studies*, 50(2): 155–170.

Jokić-Begić, N. 2010. Cognitive-behavioral Therapy and Neuroscience: Towards Closer Integration. *Psychological Topics*, 19(2): 235–254.

Kabat-Zinn, Jon. 2013. *Full Catastrophe Living Using the Wisdom of Your Body and Mind to Face Stress, Pain, and Illness*. New York: Bantam Books.

Kandel, E. R. 2006. *In Search of Memory: The Emergence of a New Science of Mind*. New York: W. W. Norton & Company.

Mayuzumi, K. 2006. The Tea Ceremony as a Decolonizing Epistemology: Healing and Japanese Women. *Journal of Transformative Education*, 4(1): 8–26.

McAlexander, T., Gershon, R., and Neitzel, R. 2015. Street-level Noise in an Urban Setting: Assessment and Contribution to Personal Exposure. *Environmental Health*, 14: 18.

Meloni, M., Müller, R., and Manusy, I. 2018. Transgenerational Epigenetic Inheritance and Social Responsibility: Perspectives from the Social Sciences. *Environmental Epigenetics*, 4(2).

Pagis, M. 2015. Evoking Equanimity: Silent Interaction Rituals in Vipassana Meditation Retreats. *Qualitative Sociology*, 38(1): 39–56.

Parkin, W. 2018. Accessed at www.theguardian.com/technology/2018/mar/04/has-dopamine-got-us-hooked-on-tech-facebook-apps-addiction.

Parkins, W., and Craig, G. 2006. *Slow Living*. Oxford: Berg.

Pederson, A., Nuetzman, E., Gubbels, J., and Hummel, L. 2018. Remembrance and Resilience: How the Bodyself Responds to Trauma. *Zygon®*, 53(4): 1018–1035.

Pfeffer, J. 2018. *Dying for a Paycheck: Why the American Way of Business Is Injurious to People and Companies*. New York, NY: HarperCollins Publishers.

Purser, R. 2015. The Myth of the Present Moment. *Mindfulness*, 6: 680–686.

Purser, R., Ng, E., and Walsh, Z. 2017. *The Promise and Perils of Corporate Mindfulness*. New York, NY: Routledge.

Simons, R., and Klopack, E. 2015. Invited Address: "The Times They Are A-Changin'" Gene Expression, Neuroplasticity, and Developmental Research. *Journal of Youth and Adolescence*, 44(3): 573–580.

Thiong'o, N. W. 2011. *Decolonising the Mind the Politics of Language in African Literature*. London, England: James Currey Ltd.

Voelker, R. 2017. Less Noise, Better Health. *JAMA*, 317(12): 1207.

Williams, W. 2005. Noise Exposure Levels from Personal Stereo Use. *International Journal of Audiology*, 44(4): 231–236.

Yellow Bird, M. 2013. Neurodecolonization: Using Mindfulness Practices to Delete the Neural Networks of Colonialism. In *For Indigenous Mind Only: A Decolonization Handbook*, edited by Waziyatawin and Yellow Bird. Santa Fe, NM: School for Advanced Research Press.

Zhang, J., Cai, W., and Lee, D. J. 1992. Occupational Hazards and Pregnancy Outcomes. *American Journal of Industrial Medicine*, 21(3): 397–408.

8 Fellow creatures

KRIS SHARES A STORY

Walking along Stinson Beach in Northern California, I watched a half dozen dogs frolicking in the surf. My own black and tan cattle dog proceeded cautiously, she was a bit anxious near the water yet wanted to socialize with the many people and dogs we passed on the beach. We came upon a smaller grey Queensland heeler and a corgi racing after a tennis ball. Their owner, a tall and strapping brown-haired man with a mustache wearing white painter's coveralls, threw the ball long with a chucker. We chatted, and he told me darkly how his dogs were rescued from Fresno, my hometown, which he described in dire terms as a broken and dangerous place filled with unwanted and abused dogs – a fact which is not untrue.

Animal rescue stories are popular in American culture and the topic of many books and films. 'Who rescued who?' declare bumper stickers adorning high-end Subarus and Toyotas. Innocent, wide-eyed dogs and cats are portrayed in television advertisements with whinging string music as a narrator intones a sinister story of cruelty and neglect by unpleasant people in even more unpleasant locales. In the eyes of my new beach acquaintance, Fresno was precisely such a place.

While pet ownership is at an all-time high in the United States, the abandonment of companion animals is a key reason for pet overpopulation. Tens of millions of stray dogs roam throughout the world There are varied reasons for the abandonment of pets, including owner illness or relocation, lack of money, a pet's old age, and behavioral problems (Coe, Young, Lambert, Dysart, Nogueira, and Rajić, 2014). According to one study, 70% of dogs and 50% of cats in the United States had been to a veterinarian in the year before their surrender, demonstrating that owners cared about their pets but perhaps did not have resources to keep them (Scarlett, 2007).

Roaming dogs are a huge problem in California's San Joaquin Valley. Stray dogs can chase children on their way to school, attack other dogs, and get hit by cars. The Fresno city animal control agency (Central California Society for the Protection of Animals) reported that it collected 18,000 stray dogs between July 2016 and July 2017; 13,000 of these dogs were euthanized, making a euthanasia rate of over 70% (Central California SPCA, 2020). By contrast, New York City shelters reported their euthanasia rates dropping from 60% in 2006 to 13% in 2016 (Newman, 2016). The San Francisco shelter reported a euthanasia rate of just 11% in the same time period (San Francisco Animal Care and Control, 2019). What makes for the huge disparity between these different places?

José Medina is an animal control officer for Fresno Humane, an agency which serves Fresno County – an area of 6000 square miles with nearly a half million residents. A talkative burly guy, José has worked for Fresno Humane since it started two years ago, when the contracted county service declared bankruptcy. He said that he drives one of four vehicles that serve a sprawling 500 square miles with 600,000 residents. Most of his day, José explained, is devoted to driving across the long country roads of Fresno County. At the shelter, he showed me kennels filled with dogs known as the 559 mix – mainly Chihuahuas and pit bull hybrids – carrying a moniker based on the local area code. Volunteers were outside packing a van with crates filled with little dogs bound for Minnesota, Oregon, and San Francisco, places where the 559 mix was welcomed.

As we started to leave the kennels and get in the truck, a rescue shelter director asked me about my research interest and said: "The key question is bonding. If we could figure out how to do that, then they would keep them. A homeless person might give food to the dog before himself, but a person who paid $1,200 for a puppy will happily give it away. How do we get them to bond?" This comment surprised me because I imagined that all of the dogs came from impoverished and crime-ridden areas of my city. I had not thought that the real heart of the issue would lie in how people construct the nature of relationships. It had not occurred to me that people who could pay a large sum of money for a pet might just as readily abandon it if they were not pleased with it. I then realized that perhaps it was really an issue that people expected to purchase a companion animal relationship in which they were the dominant 'pack leader,' intolerant of disobedience or different views on the part of the animal.

José explained to me that the biggest issues in the Valley were the lack of connection with dogs and control over one's living situation, which led to the neglect of animals. He said that he rarely encountered aggressive dogs. Poverty had an impact on animal ownership because people often lacked money for food or were evicted. Losing one's property or having to move into an apartment that did not allow dogs forced many to abandon their pets. Many in the Valley also did not know that there were places to have pets spayed or neutered for free or at low cost. Though many believe that strong cultural myths influence decisions about neutering or spaying pets, research indicates that the removal of structural barriers embedded in racial and class inequalities would be the most effective means of enhancing access to veterinary care and reducing the pet population (Decker, Camacho, Tedeschi, and Morris, 2018). José explained that when he met people with roaming dogs, he tried to talk to them about living with companion animals in the community. His biggest struggles, he said, were with people who neglected their dogs and did not walk or interact with them enough. Because they had little or no relationship with humans, these dogs were often frustrated by their confinement and behaved destructively or aggressively.

We traveled the length and breadth of the county. We visited an angry, middle-class white man in a bathrobe whose dog continuously sought to escape by jumping the fence, terrifying his elderly neighbor. He stood at his door, belligerently crossing his arms and yawningly indifferent to the travails of the older woman and his bored dog. We picked up dead chickens on the highway. We talked with concerned residents worried about a neighbor's dog. José, the resident, and the neighbors chatted in Spanish for some time and then burst into laughter when they realized that the noise they heard was the dog vocally protesting his new training regimen. The neighbors exchanged tips on animal behavior and ended the encounter by sharing pictures of their pets on their phones. Our encounters with people and animals were multifarious and diverse.

On our last call, we went to an abandoned home in the rural census-designated place of Laton, population 1,824. As we approached the house, we met another animal control officer. Neighbors had called about a litter of puppies under a house where there had been a recent eviction. The other officer had already collected the mother and father dog the previous day. Today, the officers sought to lure the puppies out from under the house. The house was in a state of disrepair, and the puppies were hiding under a house listing sharply at the foundation. Sheet metal panels lined the four sides of the house, and many were torn off. In the dark crawl space, several jacks held up the crooked house. The puppies had crawled to the middle of the house. An adolescent's American history worksheet lay nearby with an outline of 20th-century history. A coffee mug lay on the yard with a hand-printed picture of a rooster. The place felt bereft like the people had suddenly disappeared from the community just as swiftly as the puppies had appeared – the ties of relationality, care, and connection fundamentally absent for all. The day was chilly, and the wind blew the fine dust of the unkempt yard in our faces.

The animal control officers could not fit under the house where the puppies hid and had to lay flat on the ground and try to reach them; the puppies kept escaping their reach to move to the center of the house. Finally, José started banging on one side of the house, causing the remaining pups to scatter in the opposite direction. The female officer snatched up the pups as they fled. Ultimately, the officers caught all eight and placed them in the small hold of the truck, where they cowered together in a cage. We drove off, stopping only to pick up yet another dead chicken in the middle of the road on the way back to the agency.

Fresno, California, has one of the highest eviction rates in the nation (Nkosi, Crowell, Milrod, Garibay, and Werner, 2019). More than half of Fresno residents are renters, who collectively pay a high proportion of their income towards substandard housing that often has mold, bugs, lead paint, and a variety of other issues that risk the health and safety of residents. The eviction process happens fast with the vast majority of renters only one month in arrears with an over-representation of women, families, and people of color. Landlords who are often resident in other areas of the state and do not feel compelled to fix substandard housing because of the consistently high demand for low-income housing. For example, Sausalito restaurant owner Chris Henry used the rental income from his Fresno apartment complex with impunity to support his popular tavern even though his tenants faced long-term issues with heat and utility infrastructure (Johnson, 2015). Eviction has a structural impact on individual and communities by enhancing educational, health, and social disparities; increasing homelessness; and putting enormous stress on the bonds of families, communities, and mutual solidarity. It also creates trauma in individuals, families, and communities by creating housing insecurity, making life and relational bonds between people and animals ever more temporary, and severing the emotional and spiritual connection with place. Far from making choices to abandon their pets, many Fresnans were themselves blown by the winds of poverty out of the web of relationality by forces beyond their control.

I could easily see how the puppies from under the house would soon be transported to San Francisco or Minneapolis or Portland and labeled 'survivors of Fresno,' perhaps even to be delivered to the homes of people who generate rental income from the San Joaquin Valley. In these kinds of cautionary tales, so often played out on reality TV shows, the brokenness of places like the Central Valley insidiously translates into harsh judgements about the people of the region, but there are rarely analyses of the colonial structures at the root of the distress. Pet abandonment easily becomes embedded into stereotypes of social class and race, but during my time with José, I was most struck by the complexity of the role of relationality. I thought about place and kinship and what happens when we don't value our relatives.

Lessons on pathways

We live in interaction with our fellow creatures: We eat their meat, we use their skins for clothing, we work with them, and they are our companions. Our very survival as a species has long been intertwined with animals, who have served us, taught us, kept us company, and protected us. It is generally believed that humans and domesticated dogs, for example, have lived together for more than 30,000 years. Some of the earliest cave paintings depict animals, not humans, which underlines the deep-seated importance of fellow creatures. Animistic belief systems endow our fellow creatures with spiritual significance and see all living objects, such as trees, animals, humans, and ancestors, as having souls. Yet our contemporary relationships with animals are often defined by the coloniality that shapes so many aspects of our lives. Various forms of dominance and resource extraction remain the primary ways in which humans interact with animals in the Anthropocene era, from factory farming to zoos to pampered pets to trophy hunting.

We consume animals that are heavily treated with antibiotics and hormones, stressed out and abused, who obtain their water and feed from polluted sources. Though we see ourselves as being at the top of the food chain over animals, what they eat, we eat, and what they feel, we feel. And if we are able to find fresh fruits and vegetables, chances are, unless they are organic, we are ingesting various genetically modified products loaded with pesticides, herbicides, and fungicides. From food to pets to wildlife to the environment we live in, the dominant ideology of ruling over animals rather than a decolonizing approach of living in relation-ship with fellow creatures creates an imbalance in how we live, think, interact, and behave. Our many points of contact with animals often causes ill being in both ourselves and our fellow creatures.

Humans in wealthy industrialized countries are attached to pets as almost never before. The exponential rise in the number of companion animals (defined as animals primarily designated for the company or enjoyment of a household) in recent years demonstrates the increasing value people place on the human-animal relationship. People have gerbils, horses, birds, cats, fish, and a wide variety of other pets. It is estimated that there are 700 million domestic dogs and 600 million cats globally (Hughes and McDonald, 2013). With current rates of pet ownership rising sharply among the emerging middle and upper classes, pets in China are no longer considered the bourgeois luxury they were under Chair-man Mao. And in high-income regions of the world, pet ownership has increas-ingly been seen as pet parenthood.

We have play dates for dogs, take them to spas, buy toys for them, and dress them up for holidays. There are cat cafes in Amsterdam and llama treks in New Mexico, and it is possible to spend a sleepover at the Monterey Bay Aquarium with the fish. Pets are no longer seen solely as commodities to provide services but have become beloved companions. Anthropologist Donna Haraway (2015, 33) has noted,

> Commonly in the US, dogs are attributed with the capacity of 'unconditional love.' According to this belief, people, burdened with misrecognition, con-tradiction, and complexity in their relations with other human, find solace in unconditional love from their dogs. In turn, people love their dogs as chil-dren. In my opinion, both these beliefs are not only based on mistakes, if not lies, but they are also in themselves abusive – to dogs and humans.

Haraway goes on to term this limited form of relationality as "caninophiliac nar-cissm," meaning that it reduces the dogs to serving the needs of humans, thus placing them at risk of abandonment when human affection wavers or conve-nience intervenes, as the director of the rescue agency pointed out in our story. Studies show that the main reasons for animal relinquishment are aggressive companion animal behavior, housing issues, and caretaker issues (Coe, Young, Lambert, Dysart, Nogueira, and Rajić, 2014). Nonetheless, research suggests that people who have pets experience less loneliness (Novak and Sudec, 2015), have lower blood pressure (Allen, Blascovich, and Mendes, 2002), have better mental health (Walsh, 2009), and have stronger social connections (Bao and Schreer, 2016). Children raised with animals have stronger immune systems (Fall et al., 2015). Pets can also enhance social capital by building connections between strangers (Wood and Bulsara, 2005). There has been an explosion in the number of emotional support animals in recent years, reflecting new ways that people with mental health issues relate to and are comforted by the presence of fellow creatures. Our relationship to companion animals is multilayered and compli-cated, with unruly edges in our systems of oppression.

In many countries, dogs remain unconfined, and on many Indigenous lands, dogs roam and are owned by none. They are part of the whole community, as we will see in the story at the end of this chapter. Some of the complexities of living with dogs in urban settings are the needs to license them, leash them, and confine them from other humans and the dangers of roadways and other hazards. The canine nature, evident in dogs' wolf ancestor-siblings, is to wander, which does not suit our contemporary ways of living, particularly in urban settings. Consider our contradictory relationship with cats, who we view as companions and untamed, straddling the line between tame and wild. Thought to have traveled with colonial explorers who needed cats to control the rat population on ships, domestic cats have become established throughout the world as beloved pets. Yet they are also considered to be feral – dangerous because of their lack of socialization with humans and tendency to form their own self-governing colonies. Seen as bearing disease and a hazard to wild bird populations, feral cats are often targeted for destruction by health and safety officials.

Our discomfort with the binary between wild and domestic small animals reflects disturbances between social structures, relationality, and the expectations of and by companion animals. In some areas, feral cats and loose dogs are seen as a scourge – running in the streets, spreading disease, and sometimes turning aggressive towards humans. In other areas, as we shall see, a rez dog is simply living as it should. But what accounts for the difference between the beloved pets, free-roaming domestic animals, and animals seen as dangerous and at large? We do not extend the same tenderness and care towards animals not classified as pets; some animals are considered simply resources or spectacles for human use rather than sentient beings similar to us and equally worthy of our love, respect, and connection. How are these borders between the wild and domestic drawn? Our extractive capitalist social structures maintain these differences in our relationships to our fellow creatures, but what happens when the borders dissolve?

Settler colonialist ideologies brought a deeply rooted binary between man and nature that expressed itself in relation to animals through domination, settlement, and commodification. Based on Cartesian dualism, which divided all sentient beings between those seen as able to think and analyze and those that simply exist, settler colonialism created a hierarchy of being that ranked fellow creatures as unequal and secondary to human beings. The Cartesian anthropocentric view of our fellow creatures as lesser beings in the hierarchy has made possible the extractive capitalist commodification of animals through activities such as industrial farming, hunting for sport, and laboratory experimentation. As our ways of being and knowing shifted through colonization, so our ways of acting towards animals also changed.

When we consider the complexity of the San Joaquin Valley described in stories throughout this book, we can see how interconnected systems of oppression, such as environmental racism, extreme class inequalities, and health disparities, construct lines of containment that disconnect us from our fellow creatures. The Valley was once an area of foraging for Indigenous Peoples, but settler colonialists brought cattle grazing in the nineteenth century, which pushed native peoples off the land and fundamentally altered the landscape. Through the intensified process of global capitalism in the twentieth century, factory-like Concentrated Animal Feeding Operations (CAFOs) emerged as ways to mass produce meat products. CAFOs are defined by the US Department of Agriculture as farming operations where over a thousand animal units are confined at least 45 days per year (USDA, 2020). Tulare County in the San Joaquin Valley is one of the top dairy cow counties in the United States in 2007, with nearly a half million head of cattle on 244 farms worth $1.8 billion (Milk editors, 2014). CAFOs are powerful polluters that create lakes of manure, send nitrites from animal feedlots and pesticides into the soil and groundwater, and release air pollution from cow gases. The San Joaquin Valley also has a concentration of industrial broiler chicken slaughterhouses that have been sanctioned for animal cruelty, infectious disease, and pollution. All of these industries pay workers low wages, which further add to financial and housing insecurity that speeds the cycle of multispecies oppression. Animals are at the center of colonizing systems of oppression as resources to be extracted and objects of amusement and consolation, yet they are rarely centered in discussions about environmental and social justice, reinforcing anthropocentric frameworks of social change (Whitley, 2019).

Though extinction has long been part of evolution, we are now seeing animal extinction at 1,000 to 10,000 times the normal rate, with one in five species currently facing extinction and up to 99% of species in danger by the end of the century (Neuhauser, 2015). This mass extinction will have a dramatic impact on the viability of human beings on this planet, underlining the common fate that we share with all creatures. As we have discussed, settler colonialism is intertwined with a deeply rooted binary between man and nature that expresses itself in relationality to animals through domestication, settlement, and commodification. This anthropocentric framework has produced a world of domination over animals in which the lack of connection with our fellow creatures now threatens our very existence. In this chapter, we consider how we could decolonize our relationship with our fellow creatures and ways that social work practice has sought to restore our relationship through healing practices. We end with a story by Michael about rez dogs.

Decolonizing our relationship with fellow creatures

When settler Europeans first came to North America, it was said that the waters were so full of fish they had trouble navigating their ships. Passenger pigeons traveled in packs of millions so that bystanders had to run for cover or be covered with excrement. Vast herds of buffalo roamed the Great Plains. This great abundance attracted the extractive settler colonialists, who sought to conquer the territory and use the animals as resources, starting the Anthropocene era on its ecocidal logic. As Davis and Todd (2017, 763) note,

By linking the Anthropocene with colonization, it draws attention to the violence at its core, and calls for the consideration of Indigenous philosophies and processes of Indigenous self-governance as a necessary political corrective, alongside the self-determination of other communities and societies violently impacted by the white supremacist, colonial, and capitalist logics instantiated in the origins of the Anthropocene.

We start this discussion of decolonizing our relationship with fellow creatures by first exploring Indigenous kinship with fellow creatures before unpacking the logic of settler colonialism because the erasure of Indigeneity and its cosmologies has shaped all our interactions with animals since the conquest. As Indigenous scholar and member of the Driftpile Cree Nation Billy-Ray Belcourt (2014) notes, anthropocentrism, settler colonialism, and white supremacy operate hand in hand by appropriating territory for settlers and commodifying animals as products in the capitalist food chain. Attempts to liberate animals without disrupting settler colonial ideologies and systems of oppression and resource extraction continue to render Indigeneity and Indigenous ways of knowing invisible.

Abundant archaeological evidence shows that many species of animals have lived in close interaction with humans for at least 14,000 years (Serpell and Barnett, 2017). Animals have been shamans, guides, and teachers from time immemorial (Walsh, 2009). Animism, which reflects a broad spectrum of spiritualities, can be seen as a worldview that considers animals and nature as kindred spirits to human beings. Settler colonial frameworks designate humans as having consciousness and therefore superior to animals. Animists, however, see fellow creatures as living beings like humans that relate and communicate and have intentional behaviors that are not only seen through the lens of the centrality of human beings (Harvey, 2005).

Animals have had both spiritual and material significance in the lives of human beings since prehistory because humans were dependent on animals for survival. Theoretical archaeologist Dimitrij Mlekuž (2013) argues against anthropocentric views of the domestication of animals, claiming that fellow creatures were active participants in the development of pastoralism. Pointing out that living with animals is a profoundly embodied practice of commonly sustaining the needs of feeding, nurturing, watering, and sheltering, Mlekuž rejects the view of herd animals as passive and sees the development of the herd as co-constructed between animals and humans situated in their environment:

> When living close together with other species for prolonged periods they tend to bond, or create social links. Through bonding with people (and other species) humans became incorporated within animal social organization and animals became part of the power and social relations of human households. A new hybrid society emerged, consisting of humans and non-humans alike. This new set of relations between people and animals brought about a different use of caves, which in turn influenced relations between people and animals. Caves as a material culture and as special places in a landscape thus played an active role in changing relationships between people and animals

during the Neolithic. In fact, they fixed the way people and animals became a herd.

(Mlekuž, 2013, 159)

Here Mlekuž brings out the complex relationality of humans, animals, and Mother Earth. The eerie, spectral landscapes of caves have often been spaces of ritual where the nonhuman and human meet at the node between the sacred and material world (Mlekuž, 2019). A decolonizing view of relationality with animals thus departs from the view that fellow creatures and human beings have been active participants in co-constructing forms of sociality, spirituality, and living in diverse contexts. As such, animals are considered kin to humans and Mother Earth.

Traditional ecological knowledge (TEK) brings a holistic view of the interdependency and sustainability of human and animal connection that often also embodies a spiritual connection as well. Before settler colonialism, Indigenous cultures necessarily lived in close harmony with the environment and animals because of their mutual dependence for survival. The Māori of Aotearoa's strong interconnection with animals infuses tribal traditions of humans transforming into creatures such as fish and birds, which shows an intimate relationship with animals and the environment. The Arikara have an origin story that places animals equal with humans or as having formerly been human. Indigenous Peoples have had a rich and interconnected physical, emotional, and spiritual sustaining relationship between humans and animals.

Traditional ecological knowledge reflects the depth of scientific knowledge that Indigenous Peoples have had for millennia based on acute local observation. TEK has used egalitarian principles for millennia to manage the natural resources of Mother Earth sustainably and in collaboration with our fellow creatures. The relationship of humans to coyotes is a good example of the difference between TEK and settler colonial approaches. Coyote tales are prevalent and diverse among Native American tribes as the coyote occupies a singular place in North American Indigenous ceremonies and worldviews. The small canine has traditionally been a revered figure throughout North American and known for as an intelligent and crafty trickster. Though sometimes seen as a devious and malignant figure, the coyote has also been viewed as performing as a kind of Robin Hood for the people, using its cunning to benefit people, such as in the myth of giving fire to people amongst California tribes (Kerven, 2018). Speculating as to why the coyote attained such a special place in North American Indigenous spirituality, Dan Flores says,

Ten millennia ago the first Americans would have had many scores of animal candidates for their deity figures. Charismatic figures like mammoths or dire wolves or saber-toothed cats might seem to us more likely choices, and in the early stages of human settlement, perhaps they had been gods. I speculate that as the Wisconsin Ice Age gave way to a rapidly warming world, coupled with the great simplifying event known as the Pleistocene Extinctions . . . wild coyotes captured the imaginations of the Indian [*sic*] peoples of the time as creatures endowed with special abilities. I suspect that the coyote's evident skill in surviving those profound changes, when the big, charismatic species could not, attracted human attention.

(Flores, 2017, 24)

Despite the scrawny appearance of coyotes, they have been seen by Indigenous Peoples as mystical beings precisely because of their lean, adaptive qualities of survival, which larger and more powerful beasts often lack and thus become extinct.

Coyotes have appeared as mischievous trickster figures in the stories throughout many Indigenous cultures, reflecting its uncanny ability to evolve and survive in changing circumstances. Since the advent of settler colonists in North America, the coyote has been the focus of many eradication efforts by the government. Seen as a predator, there were many efforts throughout the twentieth century to kill off coyotes through poisoning, shooting, trapping, and starving. Like humans, coyotes have developed a fission–fusion adaption, which means that they are flexibly able to function both as a pack and individually. This makes coyotes singularly able to survive persecution. So, despite the many decades of efforts to eradicate and control the coyote, it remains a uniquely resilient and adaptable animal that continues to infringe on human-dominated landscapes. Coyotes are perhaps anomalous in the settler colonial world because of their ease in trespassing both in the wild and domestic worlds, confusing the lines between the two and making authorities nervous.

Western debate over the rights of animals has been fierce and contentious. Emerging with social movements of the 1960s that advocated for the rights of living things and the planet, the animal rights movement seeks to erase the moral distinction between humans and animals. Revulsion about the way animals have come to be treated through settler colonial frameworks and extractive capitalist conditions of production such as trophy hunting, fur farming, laboratory testing, and factory-produced meat gave rise to the animal liberation movement. Though individual animal cruelty is punished, a variety of 'ag gag' laws in the United States makes it difficult to expose systemic animal cruelty in slaughterhouses (Fiber-Ostrew and Lovell, 2016). Fierce political and cultural struggles have emerged over the merits and dangers of eating meat or wearing fur.

Moral philosophers (Ryder, 2000; Singer and Mason, 2006), feminists (Donovan and Adams, 2007), geographers (Yusoff, 2018), and other interdisciplinary scholars (Taylor and Twine, 2014) have been concerned with the intersectionality of oppressions and speciesism. The interdisciplinary field of critical animal studies has emerged in recent years to challenge speciesism and argue for an ethical approach to the human-animal connection, but it often does not question the settler colonial system that has constructed and maintained these hierarchies (Ulicsn, Babai, Vadász, Vadász-Besnyői, Báldi, and Molnár, 2019). Posthumanism, an emerging area of philosophical study, rejects the primacy of humanism and speciesism challenging the borders between embodied existence and other forms of being by considering what is conceptualized as human to be obsolete

(Smart and Smart, 2019). Critical humanism, according to feminist philosopher Rosi Bradiotti (2013, 28–29), aims to "further the analysis of power by developing the tools and the terminology by which we can come to terms with masculinism, racism, white superiority, the dogma of scientific reason and other socially supported systems of dominant values." The interweaving of all of these issues shows that at the heart of decolonizing our relationship with our fellow creatures is the need to unsettle anthropocentrism in all its forms.

Integrating fellow creatures in social work practice

Here we briefly explore some of the different ways that our fellow creatures have been integrated into social work practice. Social work with animals is a burgeoning field of practice, though it remains an underutilized tool in integrative healing. Western social work has long departed from an anthropocentric orientation, as we have noted earlier, and has rarely considered animals as part of its scope of activities or care. The focus on human rights and the person-in-environment framework demonstrates the centrality of people and society with an object-subject relationship in the conceptualization of well-being. Ways that we have constructed our workplaces have also made the presence of animals a health and insurance risk. Our ways of knowing and doing social work have emerged from an anthropocentric orientation.

The origins of the American Humane Society, founded to protect both children and animals, were deeply rooted in the same kinds of social reform movements that produced social work (Hoy-Gerlach, Delgado, and Sloane, 2019). Just as children were considered property in many Western industrialized countries until the twentieth century, animals continue to be labeled as property today. While children have now been recognized as embodying intrinsic rights as human beings, animals generally do not and continue to have the status of property in most societies. Our fellow creatures remain largely peripheral to social work theory and practice and are conceptualized as having value only in relation to serving human needs. Thus, social work practice often continues to view animals in therapeutic settings through the lens of settler colonialism.

In recent years, greater attention has been placed on the significance of animal-human relationships in social work, though animals have held illustrious positions in therapeutic history. Sigmund Freud regularly brought his Chow Chow, Jofi, to therapy sessions. And already in 1964, psychiatrist Boris Levinson observed that sessions with children were more beneficial when his dog was present (McClaskey, 2019, 337). Children's toys, after all, are often in the form of teddy bears and other animals. A wealth of studies have shown that companion animals support human development and provide emotional support (Purewal et al., 2017), assist with disabilities (Carlisle, Johnson, Mazurek, Bibbo, Tocco, and Cameron, 2018), develop empathy and support people with trauma (Amiot, Bastian, and Martens, 2016; Katz and Burchfield, 2018; Maharaj, 2016), and help with bereavement (Chur-Hansen, 2010).

Animal-assisted therapy has emerged as a new specialization of therapeutic practice (Geist, 2011). Encompassing any practice or intervention that uses animals in a therapeutic way to enhance well-being, animal-assisted therapy can be done with domesticated animals, such as dogs or cats, or with farm animals or marine animals. Social work interventions with animals often occur within institutions, such as prisons, old age homes, or schools but can also be on an individual basis. Service and emotional-support animals have become ubiquitous in this day and age and have a variety of purposes. Service animals, which are often dogs or miniature horses, are formally trained can help guide those with visual or aural disabilities or even recognize the signs of potential seizures or allergens. Emotional support animals can represent a wide variety of species and assist individuals with a variety of disabilities through alleviating symptoms of issues such as anxiety and depression.

Much of the research on the human-animal connection can be seen as focusing either on the physical and mental health benefits of companion animals or examining the complex harms of animal cruelty and abuse. Extensive research has documented that animal cruelty is a major predictor of interpersonal violence (Macias-Mayo, 2018). Cruelty directed towards companion animals is routine in many cases of domestic violence (Newberry, 2017). The hoarding of animals in inappropriate environments where their basic needs are not met is often indicative of socially isolated people with mental health issues (Peacock, Chur-Hansen, and Winefield, 2012). Some studies have suggested that individuals suffering from trauma may see themselves as having a 'special' relationship with animals while distrusting humans, even if they are maintaining those animals in substandard environments (Williams, 2014).

While the field of social work recognizes the value of companion animals, there is limited information about how this knowledge is taught or applied in practice (Risley-Curtiss, 2010). Social work education and practice's orientation remains anthropocentric (Risely-Curtiss, Rogge, and Kawam, 2013), but some studies shed new light. Legge (2016) discusses how animal-assisted interventions could be connected to anti-oppressive practice, and Hanarahan (2011) further explores the discriminatory nature of speciesism by implicating the anthropocentric frameworks at the core of much social work practice. Indeed, some have called for an explicit link between ecological theories of social work and animals, rejecting an anthropocentric approach to social work (Evans and Gray, 2012). The Institute for Human-Animal Connection at the University of Denver led by Philip Tedeschi is a good example of decentering anthropocentric approaches to social work knowledge through the development of animal-assisted clinical practice (Tedeschi, Fitchett, and Molidor, 2005). These types of initiatives offer integrative paths to healing.

To illustrate the contemporary complexity of human–animal understandings and to trouble notions of how care with animals is conceived, we end this story with Michael's reflections on rez dogs.

Michael's story

In the mid-1990s, when I was an assistant professor in the School of Social Welfare at the University of Kansas, I was asked by colleagues at Haskell Indian Nations University to be consultant on a Native American education study in Arizona. My job was to create the project research design and share it with the Arizona tribal leaders and staff we would be working with. During the first meeting we had with education leaders from the Gila River Pima Indian community, we discussed what the tribe was hoping to gain from our research and what we were prepared to do to make sure they were satisfied with our approach and efforts. After sharing our research plan and goals during the first part of the morning, we took a break and went outside. As we were talking, a couple of dogs trotted by. When they noticed us, they coasted to a stop, pausing briefly, sniffing in our direction, probably enticed by the smell of the pinion coffee we were drinking and doughnuts we were eating. After a few moments of uncertainty, they continued down the road and then crossed into a yard and disappeared behind one of the rez houses.

At about that moment, Gilbert, the tribal education director, asked me, "Hey, Mike, do you guys have rez dogs back home?" I smiled and answered, "Yeah, we do. Sometimes there are lot of them hanging out in the community. Sometimes you don't see that many. I think it depends on the time of the year. Back home, a lot of us rez kids grew up and hung out with rez dogs. My mom used tease my friends and I about being rez dogs. She said that because of our little fuzzy, short haircuts and raggedy, dirty clothes, she couldn't tell us kids apart from the dogs." We all laughed.

Gilbert said, "I have a rez dog story for you: Not too long ago, some inmates escaped from the Arizona State Prison in Phoenix. They were Indian guys. I guess they were picked up for vagrancy and writing bad checks. Anyway, they escaped on foot, and after weaving their way through Phoenix, they ended up crossing onto our tribal lands. The authorities couldn't figure out where they went for some time, but then finally someone reported seeing them crossing our rez. Before long, the police brought in these expensive, purebred tracking dogs and put them on the trail of these guys. They actually came right through here, where those rez dogs we were watching were just walking. When the police dogs finally tracked them into our community, our rez dogs attacked the police dogs and chased them away and so the inmates escaped. I guess you could say that rez dogs know the good guys from the bad." We all laughed and laughed. It's a story that I've never forgotten.

My mother was correct. I am a rez dog. I know the good guys from the bad. Whenever I visit tribal communities, I am always on the lookout for my relatives, the rez dogs. I want to know their stories: How did they get to where they are today? How did they survive? What happened to their babies, their parents, their friends, and their culture? What do they dream about? What hopes do they have for the future? What can they tell us about the fate of the human race and the planet? And, just like Indigenous Peoples, they have their own tribal rez dog narratives and teachings, which are embedded in our own human Indigenous histories. In the Arikara origin story, there were two sleeping dogs forgotten when the first blessings were made in the tribe. In the story, when the dogs awoke, they were distressed and said to the people: "You neglected to make your smoke offerings to us, and in punishment of your neglect, we shall follow you always." The dogs were Sickness and Death.

Rez dogs are often thought of as abandoned, stray dogs, running loose on Native American reservations in the United States and Canada. They have no human owners and are not adequately cared for, although many folks in a community may feed them and give them shelter during inclement weather. Unless you live near or on an Indian reservation, you may have never heard of them. Yet they are teachers of the past and present times. They reflect our shadow side and our better angels. When we are in balance and see that all things are sacred then we can offer the blessings of smoke so that we shall live. But as the dogs in the Arikara origin story remind us, we have short memories, we forget, we neglect, and our errors come back to bite us, never leave us, and follow us always.

Rez dogs are iconic creatures; in some respects, they are mavericks that shun human companionship, preferring the company of others in their pack. In other ways, they are symbols of survival and resilience since, not unlike Native Americans, that have had to adapt to the ravages, violence, and impositions of a colonial and postcolonial settler society. Some rez dogs have feral qualities, and so do some Indigenous Peoples. Maybe the feral dogs are the decolonized ones.

In the past, many tribes held very high regard for dogs. Dogs have accompanied and lived with humans for at least 15,000 years. It is said that dogs were the first animals to begin living with humans, sharing the fires of our ancestors and serving as companions, guards, hunters, pack animals, babysitters, and protectors. If not for dogs, it is doubtful that many human groups would have survived or dispersed as widely as we have across the planet. Dogs were often thought to be divine escorts for humans who were passing into the spirit world.

Different plains tribes in the United States derive their surnames from dogs, such as Dog Skin, Two Dogs, Spotted Dog, Red Dog, and Old Dog. The names chronicle the periods when Indigenous People chose or were given these names as a reminder of some important cultural event, story, teaching, or sacred time. Some tribes named important societies after dogs: the Crazy Dog Society of the Arikara and the Blackfeet, the Dog Soldiers of the Cheyenne, and the Dog Dancers of the Hidatsa. All of these groups featured warriors that exhibited impeccable behavior, bravery, courage, service to the people, humility, generosity, and protectors of the tribe. The connection between humans and dogs exists even at the microbial level. Recent microbiome research has revealed that humans and dogs share the same microbe communities and that dog ownership appears to reduce allergy rates among children in such households (Du, 2013).

The colonization and invasion of the 'New World' by Europeans, and later by Americans, drastically changed the cultures and lives of Indigenous Peoples. As white supremacy, death, and alien religions spread among our nations, the relationship and beliefs that we had with, and held about, dogs changed for the worse. As Indigenous languages, music, dances, cultural practices, and important societies were destroyed and banned by our colonizers, the ancient beliefs and practices that incorporated dogs into tribal life dissipated, breaking a sacred connection.

Unfortunately, in our own survival and recovery from colonization, we have forgotten the important role that dogs have had in our history and that the suffering of the settlers has compounded the suffering of Indigenous Peoples which has compounded the suffering of dogs and other fellow creatures. We must no longer think of dogs as problems, pests, or threats to our public health. Instead, we must remember that an important aspect of decolonizing our relationship with dogs and all other fellow creatures means we must restore our cultural beliefs and relationships with one another, and that when the world of dogs is out of order so is ours.

This became very clear to me when I worked with my colleagues from the Institute For Human-Animal Connection at the University of Denver in 2015 to co-sponsor a study on my reservation entitled, "Cultural restoration, humane education and addressing free roaming dog populations on Fort Berthold Reservation, North Dakota." We did several interviews with tribal members about our rez dogs and heard many compelling, heartbreaking, happy-ending, humorous, and sacred cultural stories. One of the interviews I remember most was with my younger sister Bernadine Grinnell. At the end of her interview she looked at me and leaned forward and said, "do you know why we have such strife and hardships among our people?" I shook my head no. She paused and said, "it's because we forgot how to take care of our dogs, and Michael, you know as well as I do that dogs are sacred to our people." I nodded again. "How we take care of our dogs is indicative of how healthy or sick we are and we've been sick for long time." Earlier during the interview, Bernie broke into tears as she told me how her dog, who was a companion and protector to both she and her elderly mother's (my grandmother), had recently died. About a year after her interview Bernadine passed into the spirit world. I'm sure that when she died her dog companion met her and helped her on her journey. I'm thinking that when my time comes to pass into the spirit world, my rez dog that I had as a young man will meet me and be my divine escort on my journey. Even in the spirit world there is a place for rez dogs and decolonization.

References

Allen, B., Blascovich, B., and Mendes, B. 2002. Cardiovascular Reactivity and the Presence of Pets, Friends, and Spouses: The Truth About Cats and Dogs. *Psychosomatic Medicine*, 64(5): 727–739.

Amiot, C., Bastian, B., and Martens, P. 2016. People and Companion Animals. It Takes Two to Tango. *BioScience*, 66(7): 552–560.

Bao, K., and Schreer, G. 2016. Pets and Happiness: Examining the Association Between Pet Ownership and Wellbeing. *Anthrozoos*, 29(2): 283–296.

Belcourt, B. 2014. Animal Bodies, Colonial Subjects: (Re)Locating Animality in Decolonial Thought. *Societies*, 5(1): 1–11.

Braidotti, R. 2013. *The Posthuman*. Cambridge: Polity Press.

Carlisle, G. K., Johnson, R. A., Mazurek, M., Bibbo, J. L., Tocco, F., and Cameron, G. T. 2018. Companion Animals in Families of Children with Autism Spectrum Disorder: Lessons Learned from Caregivers. *Journal of Family Social Work*, 21(4–5): 294–312.

Central California Society for the Prevention of Cruelty to Animals. 2020. *Shelter Animals Count*. Accessed 17 March 2020 at www.ccspca.com/wp-content/uploads/2018/11/Shelter-Animals-Count-2016-2017.pdf.

Chur-Hansen, A. 2010. Grief and Bereavement Issues and the Loss of a Companion Animal: People Living with a Companion Animal, Owners of Livestock, and Animal Support Workers. *Clinical Psychologist*, 14(1): 14–21.

Coe, J. B., Young, I., Lambert, K., Dysart, L., Nogueira, B. L., and Rajić, A. 2014. A Scoping Review of Published Research on the Relinquishment of Companion Animals. *Journal of Applied Animal Welfare Science*, 17(3): 253–273.

Davis, H., and Todd, Z. 2017. On the Importance of a Date, or Decolonizing the Anthropocene. *ACME*, 16(4): 761–780.

Decker Sparks, J. L., Camacho, B., Tedeschi, P., and Morris, K. N. 2018. Race and Ethnicity Are Not Primary Determinants in Utilizing Veterinary Services in Underserved Communities in the United States. *Journal of Applied Animal Welfare Science*, 21(2): 120–129.

Donovan, J., and Adams, C. J. 2007. *The Feminist Care Tradition in Animal Ethics: A Reader*. New York: Columbia University Press.

Du, X. 2013. Microbiology: Dogs and Owners Share Microbes. *Nature: International Journal of Science*, 496: 400.

Evans, N., and Gray, C. 2012. The Practice and Ethics of Animal-assisted Therapy with Children and Young People: Is It Enough that We Don't Eat our Co-workers? *British Journal of Social Work*, 42(4): 600.

Fall, T., Lundholm, C., Ortqvist, A. K., Fall, K., Fang, F., Hedhammar, A., and Almqvist, C. 2015. Early Exposure to Dogs and Farm Animals and the Risk of Childhood Asthma (Report). *JAMA Pediatrics*, 169(11): e153219.

Fiber-Ostrow, P., and Lovell, J. S. 2016. Behind a Veil of Secrecy: Animal Abuse, Factory Farms, and Ag-Gag Legislation. *Contemporary Justice Review*, 19(2): 230–249.

Flores, D. 2017. *Coyote America: A Natural and Supernatural History*. New York: Basic Books.

Geist, T. 2011. Conceptual Framework for Animal Assisted Therapy. *Child and Adolescent Social Work Journal*, 28(3): 243–256.

Hanrahan, C. 2011. Challenging Anthropocentricism in Social Work Through Ethics and Spirituality: Lessons from Studies in Human-Animal Bonds. *Journal of Religion & Spirituality in Social Work: Social Thought*, 30(3): 272–293.

Haraway, D. J. 2015. *The Companion Species Manifesto: Dogs, People, and Significant Otherness*. Chicago: Prickly Paradigm Press.

Harvey, G. 2005. *Animism: Respecting the Living World*. London: Hurst & Co.

Hoy-Gerlach, J., Delgado, M., Sloane, H., and Arkow, P. 2019. Rediscovering Connections between Animal Welfare and Human Welfare: Creating Social Work Internships at a Humane Society. *Journal of Social Work*, 19(2): 216–232.

Hughes, J., and MacDonald, D. W. 2013. A Review of the Interactions Between Free-roaming Domestic Dogs and Wildlife. *Biological Conservation*, 157: 341–351.

Johnson, B. 2015. *More Than 100 Summerset Village Tenants Filing Lawsuit Against Landlord Chris Henry*. Accessed 17 April 2019 at https://abc30.com/chris-henry-lawsuit-habitability-claim/1109196/.

Katz, N., and Burchfield, K. B. 2018. Special-Needs Companion Animals and Those Who Care for Them. *Society & Animals*, 28(1): 21–40.

Kerven, R. 2018. *Native American Myths Collected 1636–1919*. Morpeth, United Kingdom: Talking Stone.

Legge, M. M. 2016. The Role of Animal-Assisted Interventions in Anti-Oppressive Social Work Practice. *British Journal of Social Work*, 46(7): 1926–1941.

Macias-Mayo, A. 2018. The Link Between Animal Abuse and Child Abuse. *American Journal of Family Law*, 32(3): 130–136.

Maharaj, N. 2016. Companion Animals and Vulnerable Youth: Promoting Engagement between Youth and Professional Service Providers. *Journal of Loss and Trauma*, 21(4): 335–343.

McClaskey, B. 2019. Companion Animals and Their Impact on Human Lives. *Midwest Quarterly*, 60(3): 335–350.

MILK (ed.). 2014. *California Has Four of the Top Five Dairy Cow Counties*. Accessed 14 February 2020 at www.agweb.com/article/california_has_four_of_the_top_five_dairy_cow_counties__NAA_Dairy_Today_Editors.

Mlekuž, D. 2013. The Birth of the Herd. *Society & Animals*, 21(2): 150–161.

Mlekuž, D. 2019. Animate Caves and Folded Landscapes. In *Between Worlds*, edited by Lindsey Büster, Eugène Warmenbol, and Dimitrij Mlekuž. Geneva, Switzerland: Springer.

Neuhauser, A. 2015. 75 Percent of Animal Species to be Wiped Out in "Sixth Mass Extinction". *US News & World Report*, p. 1.

Newberry, M. 2017. Pets in Danger: Exploring the Link between Domestic Violence and Animal Abuse. *Aggression & Violent Behavior*, 34(May): 273–281.

Newman, A. 2016. Animal Deaths Down Amid Reforms at New York Shelters. *The New York Times*, 20 January.

Nkosi, J., Crowell, A. R., Milrod, P., Garibay, V., and Werner, A. 2019. *Evicted in Fresno: Facts for Housing Advocates*. Report Prepared on Behalf of Faith in the Valley.

Novak, S., and Sudec, J. 2015. Influence of Animals on the Quality of Life of the Elderly. *Socialno Delo*, 54(1): 31.

Peacock, J., Chur-Hansen, A., and Winefield, H. 2012. Mental Health Implications of Human Attachment to Companion Animals. *Journal of Clinical Psychology*, 68(3): 292–303.

Purewal, R., Christley, R., Kordas, K., Joinson, C., Meints, K., Gee, N., & Westgarth, C. 2017. Companion Animals and Child/ adolescent Development: A Systematic Review of the Evidence. International Journal of Environmental Research and Public Health. *The Midwest Quarterly Health*, 14(234): 1–25.

Risley-Curtiss, C. 2010. Social Work Practitioners and the Human-companion Animal Bond: A National Study. *Social Work*, 55(1): 38–46.

Risley-Curtiss, C., Rogge, M. E., and Kawam, E. 2013. Factors Affecting Social Workers Inclusion of Animals in Practice. *Social Work*, 58(2): 153–161.

Ryder, R. D. 2000. *Animal Revolution: Changing Attitudes Towards Speciesism*. Oxford: Berg.

San Francisco Animal Care and Control. 2019. *Animal Care*. Accessed 13 January 2020 at www.sfanimalcare.org/about-us/shelter-statistics/.

Scarlett, J. 2007. Are You Doing All You Can to Reduce Euthanasia of Healthy, Adoptable Pets? *Veterinary Medicine*, 102(10): 638.

Serpell, J., and Barrett, P. 2017. *The Domestic Dog: Its Evolution, Behavior and Interactions with People*. Cambridge: Cambridge University Press.

Singer, P., and Mason, J. 2006. *The Way We Eat: Why Our Food Choices Matter*. Emmaus, PA: Rodale.

Smart, A., and Smart, J. 2019. *Posthumanism*. Toronto: University of Toronto Press.

Taylor, N., and Twine, R. 2014. *The Rise of Critical Animal Studies: From the Margins to the Centre*. London: Routledge.

Tedeschi, P., Fitchett, J., and Molidor, C. 2005. The Incorporation of Animal-Assisted Interventions in Social Work Education. *Journal of Family Social Work*, 9(4): 59–77.

Ulicsni, V., Babai, D., Vadász, C., Vadász-Besnyői, V., Báldi, A., and Molnár, Z. 2019. Bridging Conservation Science and Traditional Knowledge of Wild Animals: The Need for Expert Guidance and Inclusion of Local Knowledge Holders. *AMBIO – A Journal of the Human Environment*, 48(7): 769–778.

United States Department of Agriculture (USDA). 2020. *Animal Feeding Operations*. Accessed 24 January 2020 at www.nrcs.usda.gov/wps/portal/nrcs/main/national/plantsanimals/livestock/afo/.

Walsh, F. 2009. Human-Animal Bonds I: The Relational Significance of Companion Animals. *Family Process*, 48(4): 462–480.

Whitley, C. 2019. Exploring the Place of Animals and Human-animal Relationships in Hydraulic Fracturing Discourse. *Social Sciences*, 8(2).

Williams, B. 2014. Animal Hoarding: Devastating, Complex, and Everyone's Concern. *Mental Health Practice*, 17(6): 35–39.

Wood, L., Giles-Corti, B., and Bulsara, M. 2005. The Pet Connection: Pets as a Conduit for Social Capital? *Social Science & Medicine*, 61(6): 1159–1173.

Yusoff, K. 2018. *A Billion Black Anthroposcenes or None*. Minneapolis: University of Minnesota Press.

9   Mother Earth

Decolonizing pathways that connect with our experience of our surroundings – water, creativity, movement, and contemplation, and fellow creatures – are profoundly healing activities. But all healing starts from recognizing the intrinsic rights and having respect for Mother Earth. We are entering the age of climate catastrophe due to human activities. Settler colonial extractive capitalist activities during the Anthropocene have degraded the environment and our integrative relationships with one another, our fellow creatures, and places we inhabit. As a result, we are suffering physically, psychologically, emotionally, and spiritually. Our very survival – in the deepest sense of the word – depends on changing our relationship to the planet. We may need to return to the wisdom of the past to create a sustainable future.

The field of social work often highlights the significance of human rights, but only recently have environmental rights begun to enter our professional lexicon. As human rights professionals, social workers are ethically bound to incorporate the principles of dignity, respect, integrity, and self-determination into their everyday practice with clients. But what about the place where we live? Eighty years after the ratification of the Universal Declaration of Human Rights, all life on earth faces the existential threat of extinction due to the toxic activities of extractive capitalism. Rising tides, droughts, raging wildfires, and rapidly spreading infectious disease are among the myriad signs of irreversible climate catastrophe caused by human actions. We stand at a crossroads, deciding whether we stay on the same treacherous path or embark on a course that fundamentally alters our relationship to the earth. On behalf of all the peoples and nations of earth, the People's World Conference on Climate Change and the Rights of Mother Earth hosted by Bolivia in 2010 proclaimed the Universal Declaration of the Rights of Mother Earth. Bolivia was the first country in the world to incorporate these rights into its constitution. Its preamble declares,

We, the peoples and nations of Earth:

> considering that we are all part of Mother Earth, an indivisible, living community of interrelated and interdependent beings with a common destiny;
> gratefully acknowledging that Mother Earth is the source of life, nourishment and learning and provides everything we need to live well;

recognizing that the capitalist system and all forms of depredation, exploitation, abuse and contamination have caused great destruction, degradation and disruption of Mother Earth, putting life as we know it today at risk through phenomena such as climate catastrophe;

convinced that in an interdependent living community it is not possible to recognize the rights of only human beings without causing an imbalance within Mother Earth;

affirming that to guarantee human rights it is necessary to recognize and defend the rights of Mother Earth and all beings in her and that there are existing cultures, practices and laws that do so;

conscious of the urgency of taking decisive, collective action to transform structures and systems that cause climate catastrophe and other threats to Mother Earth.

As we come to end this book, we ask: How can social work as a profession incorporate the rights of Mother Earth into everyday practice? Or rather, in the midst of climate crisis, how can we *not* center Mother Earth in all of our discussions and actions to support human well-being?

Lessons on pathways

Social work now has to be practiced under the existential threat of extinction, a menace driven by human activities. Alarming natural events are having an impact on our social systems as we enter what journalist Elizabeth Kolbert (2014) calls "the sixth extinction," a period during which humans' disruption of Mother Earth's balanced and interconnected life sustaining systems is wreaking disaster. Oceans are warming, sea levels are rising, species are going extinct, deforestation is growing, and droughts and fire seasons are intensifying, all because of climate catastrophe. There are more frequent hurricanes, heat waves, and other extreme weather events. Coastal flooding menaces hundreds of communities, such as Osaka, Japan (over five million residents), Rio de Janeiro (nearly two million residents), and New York City (nine million residents) (Holder, Kommenda, and Watts, 2017). Rising temperatures are contributing to frost-free growing seasons, changes in precipitation patterns and longer and more intense droughts and heat waves – all of which disrupts food production. Climate catastrophe is imperiling human health, animal species, and the survival of plant life. One study estimates that Chicago will have between 166 and 2,217 excess deaths per year attributable to heat waves buffeted by global warming (Peng, Bobb, Tebaldi, McDaniel, Bell, and Dominici, 2011). Another study predicts substantial climate-related changes in weight and diets, resulting in greater health risks (Springmann et al., 2016). Studies indicate that marine life and ocean ecosystems are quickly disintegrating (McCauley, Pinsky, Palumbi, Estes, Joyce, and Warner, 2015). Evidence suggests that climate catastrophe is occurring faster than previous scientific estimates (Royal Society, 2017). We are rapidly moving into an unpredictable environment guided by many of the same settler colonial paradigms that thrust us into this situation. How can we shift course? What can social work as a profession do to advocate for environmental justice and support human well-being that centers respect for Mother Earth?

We live in a world fragmented and wounded because of the impact of vast inequalities and disparities in vulnerabilities. The United States constitutes 5% of the world's population but uses nearly one-fourth of the world's fossil fuels (*Scientific American*, 2018). The 12% of the world's population residing in Western Europe and North America produces 60% of private consumption spending, while 2.8 billion people survive on less than two dollars per day (Worldwatch Institute, 2018). The average home in the United States in 38% larger than in 1975, though families are smaller (McGill, 2016). According to the Sierra Club's Dave Tilford, "A child born in the United States will create thirteen times as much ecological damage over the course of his or her lifetime than a child born in Brazil" (*Scientific American*, 2018). Environmental injustice disproportionally affects impoverished, racialized, and vulnerable communities within wealthy countries. The countries that have contributed least to climate crisis are often the one most affected.

Rising global consumption has led to a voracious appetite for mobile phones, plastic water bottles, meat, larger homes, and cheap clothing, but the real costs of these habits are inequitably borne. Some communities benefit from the vast array of consumer goods, while others struggle with the enormous environmental and human costs of their production. A mobile phone, for example, considered essential for life in the West, is composed of raw materials like tungsten, which is extracted from places like the Democratic Republic of Congo. The process of obtaining this alloy often involves child slave labor, gangs, war, and systemic environmental degradation to extract it, and then it is transported to manufacturing centers in China, where workers labor for long hours and are paid very little. The contemporary global system of extractive capitalism debases both humans and Mother Earth in distinct ways in different contexts. Social work has yet to develop and widely implement strategies that rectify these great global injustices.

Environmental disaster is the end result of extractive capitalism and settler colonial ideologies. Children of color in the United States, for example, are far more likely to be exposed to lead poisoning, air pollution, and water contamination than their white counterparts (e.g., Theppeang, Glass, Bandeen-Roche, Todd, Rohde, and Schwartz, 2008; VanDerslice, 2011) On the Gulf Coast of Louisiana, for example, 9,000 square miles of ocean is largely uninhabitable by marine life due to the agricultural waste of a major meat manufacturer (Mighty Earth, 2017). Tyson Foods, which has been accused of animal cruelty and poor conditions for workers, has also been criticized for draining groundwater and for the environmental ruin of communities. As we reap the harvest of the full-scale extractive capitalist attack on all biosystems of Mother Earth, we are bound in ever tighter circles of destructive interconnection while still clinging to the settler colonial beliefs that further extraction and growing precarity can save us. As we have noted in many of the stories in this book, there are inequities in our everyday realities: Indigenous People on reservations have trouble accessing clean and affordable water, social workers assisting suicidal callers end up with health issues because their working conditions do not allow them to move, and food deserts proliferate in many areas of the abundant agricultural San Joaquin Valley. While we often focus as social workers on state-mandated care plans to mitigate the negative personal and social outcomes of these larger systems of exploitation and distress, these traumatic landscapes sap our strength and overwhelm us. It becomes difficult to imagine other ways of living.

While many of us in social work remain wedded to gradual reform within systems, some are raising the existential questions at the heart of our contemporary condition through direct action. At the 2015 United Nations Paris Climate Change Conference, Indigenous activists attempted to take center stage, warning nations of the world that they must fundamentally change course or face environmental catastrophe. The Conference refused to hear Indigenous claims, disregarding the link between Indigenous calls for the restoration of land rights, the appropriation of resources, and climate catastrophe (Goldtooth, 2010). Paddling down the Seine River in protest of their exclusion, activists demanded that Indigenous rights be included in any climate agreement. The reluctance to associate managing climate catastrophe with toppling settler colonial paradigms of being reflects the dilemma of this existentialist challenge. We social workers should be at the forefront of these difficult discussions as agents of change, questioning and fundamentally altering the systems that we sustain.

Decolonizing social work with Mother Earth

We exist not only as minds but also as embodied beings living in and intertwined with our physical environment. Our health and well-being depend on our connection with our environment, not only for extracting resources for survival but also to receive the emotional and spiritual healing that reciprocity with Mother Earth brings. Settler colonial ideologies of nature have often been replicated in social work theory and practice, but decolonizing methods are increasingly challenging anthropocentrism in social work theory and practice and offer us hope to save the planet.

Settler colonialism is based on a binary understanding of the universe that divides the mind from the body, the material from the sacred, the human from nature. For Indigenous Peoples, the sacred has always been reflected in the inherent relationality and interconnection of human beings and Mother Earth. Indigenous ways of knowing are inherently holistic, grounded in reciprocal relationships between land and people with a strong emphasis on local knowledge. As scholars Nathalie Kermoal and Isabel Altamirano-Jimenez note (2016, 8), "Indigenous knowledge is not fragmented into silos or categories; rather, ontologies, epistemologies, and experiences are interwoven into the system." Indigenous knowledge is therefore not unscientific, as evidenced by increasing scientific interest in Indigenous knowledge of local environments, but rather embodies a relational worldview. The complex appreciation of the interconnection between humans and their land is one of the key elements of Indigenous being and knowing. An Indigenous perspective goes beyond simply seeking practical solutions to the grave climate crisis in which we currently find ourselves. It calls for a fundamental realignment in our relationship to Mother Earth and the displacement of Western anthropocentrism and recognizes the inherent value and rights of streams, mountains, and other natural habitat to exist. This perspective can be seen in New Zealand's recent legislation conferring legal rights of personhood on the Whanganui River (Liu, 2017).

Early social work saw the role of the environment, land, or place from a settler colonial perspective. In the nineteenth century, the Industrial Revolution was in full force, with a colossal extraction of resources globally. Iron and coal were needed to fuel expanding factories and cities, while waterways were constructed to transport goods. Nature was either romantically constructed as a sublime pastoral landscape or as uninhabited wilderness, given only a passive role as a background canvas to humans' awe and longing for spiritual transformation. These anthropocentric perspectives create "a dehistoricized space in which the erasure of the histories of human habitation, ecological alteration, and native genocide that preceded its 'wild' valorization is, literally, naturalized" (Outka, 2008, 2). After the settler colonial genocide of native populations and the establishment of agriculture over formerly pristine nature often by enslaved labor, an Edenic pastoral was evoked that represented longing for spiritual transcendence by a colonial beholder.

Early social work in nineteenth-century North America adopted various practices of sending urban children out to the countryside. The *Toronto Star*'s and New York City's Fresh Air Fund were two prominent programs that regularly sponsored country visits starting in the late 1800s. These practices were generally framed in the narrative of transcendentalism, in which nature was viewed as providing moral uplift to impoverished children from unsanitary and vice-ridden surroundings (Cox, 2015). As geographers Mackintosh and Anderson (2009) noted,

> the beauty of nature, the hygiene of fresh air, and the antiurbanism of bourgeois reformers combined with a simple environmentalism. This created the irrational expectation that "nature" could convert the antibourgeois behavior of poor children, disadvantaged by geographies of heat, smoke, and smell, into the respectable demeanor of their Anglo-Canadian "betters."

In the United States, pristine nature, devoid of Indigenous inhabitants, was seen as a moral space that would civilize and edify youth corrupted by the poverty and criminality of their urban industrialized environments.

While some youth were taken for short visits to the countryside by various charities, many other urban European American youth were resettled with rural families. The Children's Aid Society transported foundlings and children without parents to the western regions of the United States, Canada, and Indian Territories to be adopted by settler families on what were termed 'orphan trains' in the late nineteenth century. Living with the settler families was thought to inculcate moral values in children from the city streets. These transports reduced child homelessness in urban centers on the Eastern Seaboard, delivered child farm laborers to the settlers on the frontier, and bolstered white settler colonial culture on stolen lands – all with the belief that agrarian life would morally transform street urchins. Over 200,000 children were sent on orphan trains, which started the long tradition of fostering in American child welfare (Chiodo and Meliza, 2014). Early social work interventions with nature were thus built on a hierarchy of settler colonial domination of the colonized and their land as well as an anthropocentric view of the land itself.

Nature is increasingly featuring in social work theory and practice in the form of environmental justice. The modern-day Western environmental movement was born with the publication of Rachel Carson's *Silent Spring* (1962), which documented the devastating impact of chemical and pesticide use on the land and wildlife. At the same time, there was a growing chorus of critique of the social institutions, knowledge systems, and social work methods to address conditions of late capitalism (e.g., Goodman, 1960; Reisch and Andrews, 2001). Counter-culture historian Theodore Roszak (1969) developed the concept of ecopsychology as a nature-based means to address the alienation and emptiness of modern life. Ecopsychology built on sources as diverse as Jungian archetypes, Indigenous ritualistic practices, and environmentalism to challenge dominant clinical practice and liberate people from the constraints of living in contemporary extractive capitalism (Fisher and Abram, 2002). These theories and practices drew on the rich critical traditions in the human sciences to construct new ways of practice. In the past thirty years, social work began expanding its repertoire to bring practices such as wilderness therapy for people with substance abuse issues (Bettman, Russell, and Parry, 2013), nature therapy using multifarious methods (Berger, 2010), and forest bathing (Hansen, Jones, and Tocchini, 2017) ever more into the mainstream.

As climate catastrophe has become an acute issue, social workers have grappled with ways to address the environment in policy, practice, and curriculum. One of the first articles to explicitly draw the line between social work practice and the destruction of the environment was "Habitat Destruction Syndrome" (Berger, 1995), which argued that social workers have an obligation to act to protect the environment. In 2009, the US National Association of Social Workers issued an environment policy, and in 2015 the Council of Social Work Education (CSWE, 2015) incorporated environmental justice into its educational competencies. *Environmental Social Work* (Gray, Coates, and Hetherington, 2013), for example, focuses on how to implement concrete changes in social work by considering multifaceted international approaches to environmentally sustainable practices through an ecosystems perspective.

While climate catastrophe has clearly generated greater interest in environmental issues in social work, there is a noticeable gap in the application of environmental social work methods to everyday institutional practices. How do child welfare workers and medical social workers, for example, use an environmental perspective in their daily routine and interaction with clients? There is also a broad spectrum of environmental social work concepts ranging from ecofeminism to spiritual social work to sustainable practices. Exploratory environmental social work methods have sought ways to creatively incorporate natural world from integrating environmental concepts into social work curriculum (Kemp, 2011) and enhancing professional dialogue (Coates and Besthorn, 2010). However, fundamental tensions arise between those who believe in working within the system to achieve change and those who feel there must be a radical realignment of systems.

Deep ecology, an environmental philosophy that sees all life as equally valuable, arose in a multitude of forms in the 1970s through the work of Norwegian philosopher Arne Naess, the poetry of Gary Snyder, and social movements such as ecofeminism, which sought to decenter patriarchal Western rationalism with a holistic feminist ethos. Deep ecology rejects anthropocentrism and "extends the concept of self to encompass a deep interconnectedness with all individuals, by which they mean both people and the whole of nature" (Besthorn, 2012, 61). Deep ecology therefore calls for cultivating a more authentic and deeply relational sense of self with all living things. Deep ecology is holistic and engages with the value of justice on an essential level beyond simply the social environment. Indeed, deep ecology calls for transformative ways of thinking about social work because human beings live in interconnected social and natural environments. While deep ecology incorporates a rejection of anthropocentrism and a recalibration of values, social work practice with Mother Earth must also confront the legacy of settler colonialism. Decolonizing methodologies require a radical change in the way we live with Mother Earth and one another, which starts from recognizing the legacy of Indigenous genocide and colonial conquest. Overcoming settler colonialism calls for a critical consciousness of the damage done by extractive capitalism and the restoration of many cultural beliefs and practices of the original people.

Forest therapy as indigenous social work

KRIS TELLS A STORY

Driving on Ounastie, a divided highway that crosses over the northwestern region of Finland, one passes through Enontekiö, a sparsely populated municipality of approximately 2,000 residents spread over 3,200 square miles that border Norway and Sweden. The town of Hetta consists of a few hotels for tourists, some squat brick municipal office buildings, a couple of grocery stores, the state-run liquor store Alko, a sausage kiosk, and a red-roofed brick-and-concrete Lutheran church with a slender tower. The hotels cater to tourists looking for a holiday involving cross-country skiing, trekking, or dog sledding. Like much of Sápmi, which stretches across the very far north of Europe, the landscape is flat with few trees or plants and framed by gently rolling fells that rise above the timber line. There are only two inhabitants per square kilometer in Finnish Sápmi. Three hundred miles north of the Arctic Circle, Enontekiö has a harsh climate with temperatures that fall into the double digits below zero during the long, dark winters.

Enontekiö is in Indigenous Sámi territory, an area that stretches from Kola Peninsula in Russia to Norway and is related to Indigenous communities clustered around the Arctic. When Nordic people first came to Sápmi in the fifteenth century, they forced Sámi people to convert to Christianity, forbade the traditional use of drums and *joiks*, and colonized the collective land of Sápmi. The incursion into the Finnish state after Second World War reinforced settler colonial ideologies and discriminatory practices in the everyday lives of Indigenous Peoples, which altered traditional lifeways, interrupted the traditional routes of nomadic reindeer, and depleted precious natural resources. The advent of boarding schools separated children and community, interrupting the transmission of cultural norms and ways. All of the changes have had a strong impact on the traditional Sámi subsistence economy and cultural connection with nature. These challenges have often placed Indigenous Sámi people at a disadvantage in contemporary neoliberal society, disrupting the communal bonds of the community and narrowing opportunities and choices.

The Sámi people have lived in Sápmi since the last Ice Age and have traditionally maintained a deep and abiding connection with reindeer, an animal that has provided subsistence, partnership, a rhythm to life, and spiritual inspiration to the Sámi people. The reindeer and Sámi have lived deeply intertwined lives in terms of survival and spirituality. Some of the earliest images carved on stone in Northern Europe and Asia represent reindeer, often portrayed as flying through the air (Vitebsky, 2005). These carvings suggest the marking of a cosmic landscape where sacred shamanic rituals and ceremonies were performed (Helskog, 1999). Traditionally, the Sámi have been animists, meaning that their worldviews and lifeways are not constructed on Cartesian dualism but are expansively respectful and inclusive of all living beings.

Drums have been commonly used in many Indigenous cultures, especially during rituals and ceremonies. Sámi have used sacred drums passed down for generations to prophecy, to solicit advice for the community, to reveal the best hunting and fishing places, and for ecstatic entrancement into the spirit world where shamans could help people travel to the spirit world (Joy, 2014). When settler colonial Christian missionaries came into Sámi territory in the seventeenth century, they were obsessed with sacred drums, confiscating and burning many of them and persecuting Sámi who continued to use drums, even threatening the death penalty. Sámi people were put on trial for sorcery and witchcraft for traditional practices, but as North Sámi historian and academic Veli-Pekka Lehtola points out: "The intent of Christian priests seems to have been the complete destruction of the old worldview, not just the shamanic practices" (Lehtola, 2002, 28). Today, many Sámi sacred drums can be found in European museums, which have yet to return them to their rightful place.

Sámi people were initially hunter-gatherers subsisting on a diet of berries, fish, and game (Bjørklund, 1990). Some have suggested that the gradual encroachment of Christian Nordic society on Sámi lands starting in the Middle Ages led to changes in how the Sámi worked with reindeer (Weinstock, 2013). About 1,000 years ago, the Sámi abandoned a hunter-gatherer lifestyle for nomadic pastoralism, moving with the clan's reindeer herd as it sought grazing lands. Sámi managed their natural resources through a *siida*, or local community group often composed largely of extended relatives. Sámi families moved with their herds during a yearly cycle while camping in a *lavvu*, a temporary structure similar to an Indigenous American tipi. Reindeer herding involved the entire family, and each clan member had a role to play to maintain survival in the harsh climate of the Arctic The use of the *siida* system meant that Sámi pastoralists collaborated to ensure that land was not overgrazed "through a culturally designed distributive institution, thereby regulating the carrying capacity of the pastures. The conventional view recognizes only the herder's capacity as harvester, and not as mediator. But herders constitute management units which mediate the relation between herds and pasture within a cultural framework implying strategies, negotiations, rules and sanctions" (Bjørklund, 1990, 83). Cooperation and inclusion were therefore at the heart of Sámi life in the unforgiving conditions of Sápmi.

A great deal of geopolitical and economic interest is currently focused on the Arctic. Many see it as the last strategic outpost open for exploitation as China, Russia, the United States, and the European Union compete for dominance, especially in regard to the abundant energy resources. Nordic governments have a strategic plan to build an Arctic railway to enhance mining, logging, and energy extraction. Sámi people fear that the proposed railway would decimate nomadic reindeer herds and lead to the corporate looting of Sámi homelands. The rapid environmental changes in the far north has shown that the Arctic is, in many ways, the canary in the coalmine for climate crisis.

I arrived in Enontekiö in March of 2016 after inviting myself to shadow two Sámi social workers. I went to their local red brick municipal building, where I was introduced to the staff. The main social Sámi social worker, Anne-Maria Näkkäläjärvi, wearing outdoor winter clothing, entered the coffee room briskly. She sized me up and said that we would travel north with her colleague, Ellen-Anne Labba, and a young social work intern from the University of Lapland to learn more about the everyday life of a social worker in Enontekiö. Anne-Maria, the intern, and I exited from the side door, and I tried not to lose my balance in the icy parking lot while the others strode purposefully to the municipal Fiat.

We drove for a few miles and then stopped on a side road where Ellen, slight with dark woolly clothing, emerged from a snowy landscape and climbed in the back. We then drove two hours along frozen roads with sweeping tundra vistas toward the Norwegian border. The ride was largely quiet, except for the click of Ellen's knitting needles in the back seat. The silence felt pregnant with curiosity, but I didn't want to chatter in English. I wasn't sure who these folks were or where we were going, but I trusted them as my guides. We eventually stopped at a cabin maintained for municipal workers traveling on business. Anne-Maria explained that social workers often operated on a weekly circuit, visiting various clients and Sámi elders. Due to the vastness of the landscape and the sparse population, some elders had only a weekly visit from social workers and had to survive on their own otherwise. Anne-Maria laughed about the gallons of coffee and sweet pastries that she had to consume during these visits, which often took place around the kitchen table.

We worked together to prepare the evening meal and started the sauna oven fire. Sauna is a peculiarly Finnish practice – silent and spare, it is a place of spiritual cleansing and recharge where you sweat out all of the toxins in your body and emerge refreshed. After sauna, we made a dinner of reindeer meat, rye bread, potatoes, and herring. As we ate, my hosts explained how Sámi people had always lived according to the seasonal rhythms of the reindeer. However, with the introduction and rapid growth of private property and extractive capitalist ways of life, this traditional communal lifestyle was becoming increasingly difficult to maintain.

Nordic colonial rule was first extended by Swedish missionaries who enforced Christianity on the animistic Sámi, wiping out a great deal of Indigenous artifacts. Settlers from the south have been coming north as settlers and representatives of the forest industry since the eighteenth century, but Sápmi fundamentally changed after the Second World War, when the retreating German army devastated infrastructure. The reorganization of society in Sápmi by the Finnish state included building roads across reindeer migration routes, installing Sámi people in permanent housing, placing Sámi children in boarding schools where they were required to lose their language and erase their culture, and pushing an ideology of self-hating assimilation into Finnish society.

As social workers, Anna-Maria and Ellen pointed out that many of the social and personal issues their clients struggle with are related to the ideology of settler colonialism, which has brought about a fundamentally altered relationship between the Sámi people and nature. Traditional reindeer herding becomes problematic when people seek to individualize, privatize, and grow their own profits, sometimes at the expense of others. Disputes over land use flare. Reindeer can no longer move freely when there is private property. Young people cannot afford to go into reindeer herding when they need to purchase expensive equipment, such as snowmobiles. Traditional ways of life and social connections crumble amid the onslaught of privatization. Anna-Maria pointed out that there were new calls to raise reindeer like cattle, meaning that they would be farmed as domesticated animals with different diets than they enjoyed as nomadic grazers in their natural habitat. She went on to say that the meat of farmed reindeer is fattier than that of the nomadic reindeer and not as healthy. Increased dependence on the money economy has also led to reindeer herding as an exotic and seasonal tourist activity, making the maintenance of traditional ways even more difficult. As the *siida* has collapsed, society has become more atomized, and many of the young Sámi move south in search of work, leaving elders and others behind. Sámi reindeer culture has always been based on the notion that that everyone in the community has to pitch in and that each person has a strength and something to contribute. Settler colonialism has brought an ideology of control, domination, and materialism to a place where relationality with one another and the extreme environment has always been the key to survival. The ill-being of so many, the social workers said, is related to the 'colonial wound' that disenfranchised Sámi people experience in their separation from their traditional ways of life and land.

Stereotypes of excessive alcoholism among the Sámi have had a pervasive presence in Finnish cultural representations in the media, even in the context of notoriously heavy Finnish drinking habits. Similar to demeaning depictions of Indigenous Peoples in many other parts of the world, alcoholism has often been portrayed as an essential attribute of Sámi people. One study, however, found that Sámi youth drink less than their non-Sámi counterparts, and the Arctic Indigenous most disconnected to their culture are at higher risk of excessive drinking (Spein, 2008). There are many theories of addiction, including genetic and social learning perspectives (Lebowitz and Applebaum, 2017; Preston and Goodfellow, 2006). However, cultural trauma is increasingly viewed as a key risk factor for addiction (Garcia, 2010). How can interventions enmeshed in the structural arrangements of the dominant settler colonial society help those assuaging cultural trauma through substance misuse?

In 2009, Sámi social worker Anne-Maria Näkkäläjärvi and Sámi community worker Ellen-Anne Labba received a small grant to develop *mettäterapia* (forest therapy) in their region. Forest therapy was initiated when many Sámi social workers noted that mainstream services did not address the needs of Indigenous People. The closest clinic, a large institution, is in Rovaniemi – nearly five hours away by bus – which deepens the social isolation of Sámi people with addiction issues. Clinics serving people with addiction issues offer treatment that is sometimes culturally inappropriate and does not take into account the specific cultural needs of Sámi people. Many of the concepts and words used in mainstream Finnish addiction treatment do not have equivalents in the Sámi language or worldview. Using a model of "cultural safety," Näkkäläjärvi and Labba sought to create a space for local Sámi people to heal. The framework of cultural safety emerged from Aotearoa/New Zealand in the 1980s as practitioners sought to decolonize services by reconceiving social and health services from an Indigenous perspective (Christensen, 2016).

Forest therapy is based on the idea that humans' interconnection with nature is a fundamental element of life and is healing. This is especially true for the nomadic Sámi people, who have always lived in nature. Näkkäläjärvi and Labba felt that life becomes out of balance when we lose that fundamental connection. As one of the characteristics of substance misuse is isolation and disconnection, Näkkäläjärvi and Labba thought that restoring this connection was one of the first steps toward healing. Forest therapy specifically uses Sámi concepts of health and wellness with Sámi social workers.

Starting in the summer of 2010, Näkkäläjärvi and Labba began the first forest therapy excursion. They took a handful of Sámi men out on a lake, where they stayed in a cabin and camped for several days. During the day, they participated in various traditional hunting and fishing activities. The men developed a strong group identity during this time, developing social ties, a stronger sense of self-esteem, and self-understanding. The men also reconnected with traditional Sámi folkways. The aim of the program is to help disaffected people establish a community because family has often cut them off and they are lonely. They seek to support healthy relationships and empower participants. By reconnecting people with their Indigenous ties to nature and their community, forest therapy intends to end the isolation underlying substance abuse. In being together, the participants can develop trust to talk about what is really going on and plan for the recovery process. While fishing, rowing, hiking, and preparing food, the participants work together. Forest therapy brings the elements of nature and collectivity back into their lives.

During the evening discussions, social workers help participants map their family networks, unlock the role of friends and their values, and together consider paths of change. The participants think about their lives and how to achieve their dreams. Reconnecting with nature gives participants strength, peace, safety, and relationship; it brings meaning to life. Participants report feeling less lonely and more hopeful.

Forest therapy has brought a resurgence of interest in traditional Sámi activities of hunting and fishing. People are skilled in living in nature in the north. They know how to use a compass, to fish, to forage, and to herd reindeer. The reconnection with nature that forest therapy provides opens an avenue for men to stop drinking and find new hobbies instead of returning to old drinking buddies. It's the small moments, Ellen-Anne Labba noted, of making food together, for example, that bring joy and a sense of connection. Participants felt that they could talk about their concerns in a safe place and change their thoughts about drinking. It ignites a process of change and a new motivation in life.

My visit ended with the local celebration of St. Marian's Day. I watched reindeer racing, received a gift of five pairs of fingerless gloves from a Sámi vendor, and spent an evening at a music event. We sat in a beautiful wooden room surrounded by large windows facing a luminous landscape of snow, blue in the winter light. People came dressed in traditional Sámi clothing featuring bright contrasting colors with heavy embroidery and tin ornaments. All of the clothing colors and decorations had significance that stretched back generations. Various local groups of vocalists mounted the small stage, singing Sámi songs. Niko Valkeapää, a local Sámi singer and musician, brought a blend of contemporary jazz and traditional *joiks*, haunting and evocative chants believed to be given to the Sámi people by elves and fairies thousands of years ago. There was a palpable sense of unity in the room as the music enveloped people in its power, dissolving the division between the snowy landscape outside and the warm communal gathering inside.

References

Berger, R. 1995. Habitat Destruction Syndrome. *Social Work*, 40(4): 441–443.

Berger, R. 2010. Nature Therapy: Thoughts about the Limitations of Practice. *Journal of Humanistic Psychology*, 50(1): 65–76.

Besthorn, F. 2012. Deep Ecology's Contributions to Social Work: A Ten-Year. Retrospective. *International Journal of Social Welfare*, 21(3): 248-259.

Bettmann, J., Russell, E., and Parry, K. 2013. How Substance Abuse Recovery Skills, Readiness to Change and Symptom Reduction Impact Change Processes in Wilderness Therapy Participants. *Journal of Child and Family Studies*, 22: 1039–1050.

Bjørklund, I. 1990. Sámi Reindeer Pastoralism as an Indigenous Resource Management System in Northern Norway: A Contribution to the Common Property Debate. *Development and Change*, 21(1): 75–86.

Carson, R. 1962. *Silent Spring*. New York: Houghton Mifflin.

Chiodo, J. J., and Meliza, E. 2014. Orphan Trains: Teaching about an Early Twentieth-Century Social Experiment. *Social Studies*, 105(3): 145–157.

Christensen, J. 2016. Indigenous Housing and Health in the Canadian North: Revisiting Cultural Safety. *Health and Place*, 40: 83–90.

Coates, J., and Besthorn, F. H. 2010. Building Bridges and Crossing Boundaries: Dialogues in Professional Helping. *Critical Social Work*, 11(3): 1–7.

Cox, A. 2015. Fresh Air Funds and Functional Families: The Enduring Politics of Race, Family, and Place in Juvenile Justice Reform. *Theoretical Criminology*, 19(4): 554–570.

CSWE. 2015. *Educational, Policy and Accreditation Standards*. Accessed at www.cswe.org/getattachment/Accreditation/Accreditation-Process/2015-EPAS/2015EPAS_Web_FINAL.pdf.aspx.

Fisher, A., and Abram, D. 2002. *Radical Ecopsychology: Psychology in the Service of Life*. SUNY Series in Radical Social and Political Theory. Albany: State University of New York Press.

Garcia, A. 2010. *The Pastoral Clinic: Addiction and Dispossession Along the Rio Grande*. Berkeley: University of California Press.

Goldtooth, T. B. K. 2010. The State of Indigenous America Series: Earth Mother, Piñons, and Apple Pie. *Wicazo Sa Review*, 25(2): 11–28.

Goodman, P. 1960. *Growing Up Absurd: Problems of Youth in the Organized System*. Vintage Political Science and Social Criticism 32. New York: Random House.

Gray, M., Coates, J., and Hetherington, T. 2013. *Environmental Social Work*. Milton Park, Abingdon, Oxon: Routledge.

Hansen, M., Jones, R., and Tocchini, K. 2017. Shinrin-Yoku (Forest Bathing) and Nature Therapy: A State-of-the-Art Review. *International Journal*.

Helskog, K. 1999. The Shore Connection: Cognitive Landscape and Communication with Rock Carvings in Northernmost Europe. *Norwegian Archaeological Review*, 32(2): 73–94.

Holder, J., Niko, K., and Watts, J. 2017. The Three-Degree World: The Cities That Will Be Drowned by Global Warming. *Guardian*. Accessed at www.theguardian.com/cities/ng-interactive/2017/nov/03/three-degree-world-cities-drowned-global-warming.

Joy, F. 2014. To All Our Relations: Evidence of Sámi Involvement in the Creation of Rock Paintings in Finland. *Polar Record*, 50(1): 108–111.

Kemp, S. P. 2011. Recentring Environment in Social Work Practice: Necessity, Opportunity, Challenge. *British Journal of Social Work*, 41(6): 1198–1210.

Kermoal, N. J., and Altamirano-Jiménez, I. 2016. *Living on the Land: Indigenous Women's Understanding of Place*. Edmonton: Athabasca University Press.

Kolbert, E. 2014. *The Sixth Extinction: An Unnatural History*. New York: Henry Holt.

Lebowitz, M., and Appelbaum, P. 2017. Beneficial and Detrimental Effects of Genetic Explanations for Addiction. *International Journal of Social Psychiatry*, 63(8): 717–723.

Lehtola, V.-P. 2002. *The Sámi People: Tradition in Transition*. Aanar-Inari: Kustannus-Puntsi.

Liu, K. 2017. New Zealand's Whanganui River Has Been Granted the Same Legal Rights as a Person. *Time*. Accessed at http://time.com/4703251/new-zealand-whanganui-river-wanganui-rights/.

Mackintosh, P., and Anderson, R. 2009. The Toronto Star Fresh Air Fund: Transcendental Rescue in a Modern City, 1900–1915. *Geographical Review*, 99(4): 539–562.

McCauley, D., Pinsky, M., Palumbi, S., Estes, J., Joyce, F., and Warner, R. 2015. Marine Defaunation: Animal Loss in the Global Ocean. *Science*, 347: 6219.

McGill, A. 2016. The Shrinking of the American Lawn: As Houses Have Gotten Bigger, Yard Sizes Have Receded. What Gives? *The Atlantic*. Accessed 14 March 2020 at www.theatlantic.com/business/archive/2016/07/lawns-census-bigger-homes-smaller-lots/489590/.

Mighty Earth. 2017. *New Investigation Identifies Companies Responsible for Massive Dead Zone in Gulf of Mexico*. Accessed at www.mightyearth.org/heartlanddestruction/.

Outka, P. 2008. *Race and Nature from Transcendentalism to the Harlem Renaissance*. New York: Palgrave Macmillan.

Peng, R., Bobb, J., Tebaldi, C., McDaniel, L., Bell, M., and Dominici, F. 2011. Toward a Quantitative Estimate of Future Heat Wave Mortality under Global Climate Change. *Environmental Health Perspectives*, 119(5): 701–706.

Preston, P., and Goodfellow, M. 2006. Cohort Comparisons: Social Learning Explanations for Alcohol Use among Adolescents and Older Adults. *Addictive Behaviors*, 31(12): 2268–2283.

Reisch, M., and Andrews, J. 2001. *The Road Not Taken: A History of Radical Social Work in the United States*. Philadelphia: Brunner-Routledge.

Roszak, T. 1969. *The Making of a Counter Culture: Reflections on the Technocratic Society and Its Youthful Opposition*. Garden City, NY: Anchor Books.

Royal Society. 2017. *Climate Updates: What Have We Learnt since the IPCC Fifth Assessment Report*? Accessed at https://royalsociety.org/~/media/policy/Publications/2017/27-11-2017-Climate-change-updates-report.pdf.

Scientific American. 2018. Use It and Lose It: The Outsize Effect of US Consumption on the Environment. Accessed at www.scientificamerican.com/article/american-consumption-habits/.

Spein, A. 2008. Substance Use among Young Indigenous Sami – A Summary of Findings from the North Norwegian Youth Study. *International Journal of Circumpolar Health*, 67(1): 124–136.

Springmann, M., Masons-D'Croz, D., Robinson, S., Garnett, T., Charles, H., Godfray, J., Gollin, D., Raynor, M., Ballon, P., and Scarboroughr, P. 2016. Global and Regional Health Effects of Future Food Production under Climate Change: A Modelling Study. *The Lancet*, 387(10031): 1937–1946.

Theppeang, K., Glass, T., Bandeen-Roche, K., Todd, A., Rohde, C., and Schwartz, B. 2008. Gender and Race/Ethnicity Differences in Lead Dose Biomarkers. *American Journal of Public Health*, 98(7): 1248–1255.

VanDerslice, J. 2011. Drinking Water Infrastructure and Environmental Disparities: Evidence and Methodological Considerations. *American Journal of Public Health*, 101: S109–S114.

Vitebsky, P. 2005. *The Reindeer People: Living with Animals and Spirits in Siberia*. Boston: Houghton Mifflin.

Weinstock, J. 2013. Assimilation of the Sámi: Its Unforeseen Effects on the Majority Populations of Scandinavia. *Scandinavian Studies*, 85(4): 411–430.

Worldwatch Institute. 2018. *The State of Consumption Today*. Accessed at www.worldwatch.org/node/810.

Epilogue
Dreaming a decolonized futurity

This book is going to press in the midst of the COVID-19 virus global pandemic and historic protests around the world against the colonial structures of systemic racism. The world has ground to a halt, and hundreds of thousands have died, while healthcare and social systems groan under the strain of need. Pandemics are clear barometers that brutally reveal the inequalities and ill-being at the heart of our societies. While the situation is changing every day, we feel a deep sense of sadness and horror at the suffering enveloping humanity but we feel hopeful at the promise of social transformation demonstrated by the mass of people taking to the streets saying "no more." More than ever, the pandemic reveals how fundamentally interconnected we are and the burning need for social solidarity across borders to care for one another in true relationality. And we ask: How can we reconstruct societies after COVID-19 that do not reproduce the same colonized structures and practices that we have just discussed in this book? How do we, as Arundhati Roy has pondered, pass through the portal of the pandemic? We can, as Roy observes, "choose to walk through it, dragging the carcasses of our prejudice and hatred, our avarice, our data banks and dead ideas, our dead rivers and smoky skies behind us. Or we can walk through lightly, with little luggage, ready to imagine another world. And ready to fight for it" (Roy, 2020). The many hundreds of thousands who have showed up to protest indicates that many are ready to fight for another world.

Dreaming a new world is essential to nurturing our spirit and hope that our myriad actions and mindful transformations can create a decolonized future. Maryan Abdulkarim, a Finnish author, artist, and social justice activist, has been conducting collective dreaming sessions with her self-described friend, colleague, and co-conspirator, Sonya Lindfors, a Finnish choreographer and artistic director. They see these sessions as a means of unlearning our colonized conditioning by imagining an alternative reality. Imagining and dreaming is key to acting to forge a different future.

We are deeply entwined with the legacy of our past and hopes for our future in how we understand and imagine how to change our present. Black Quantum Futurism (BQF) is a set of theoretical frameworks and practices developed by a collective facilitated by Moor Mother Goddess and Rasheedah Phillips that has developed the notion of chronological integration as a way of liberating our colonized societies. Rooted in quantum physics, African cultural traditions, and the Black experience, past and present, BQF complicates notions of time as an eternally linear and unidirectional future. BQF views time as multidimensional, with rhythms and patterns similar to Mother Earth and challenges Eurocentric notions of time as sequential, understanding the past, present, and future as relational. In rejecting a model of time as linear and teleological, inevitably leading humanity toward a progressively better future, BQF embraces memory work and illustrates how the past lives in the present and future.

Dismantling the master's time clock, in the words of Phillips, and acknowledging the circular nature of time, means recognizing the significance of past trauma in the present (Phillips, 2016). We are living the past in the present when we consider how the deep consequences of land theft, genocide, and slavery sustain colonial and historical trauma are manifested through addiction, suicide, and other self-harming behaviors in communities. Through memory work, we can recall the resilience of communities to survive demonstrating the strength of ancestral wisdom and fortitude. Acknowledging the past and making restitution through reparations, such as the restoration of land rights and correcting historical narratives, is a tangible act of hope that it builds a more just and inclusive future. Through the practices of future visioning, future altering, and future manifestation, BQF opens up the possibilities for decolonizing social change.

In a discussion of Black feminism, Tina Campt points out that futurity is more than hope – though that is important, too. Futurity is

> a grammar of possibility that moves beyond a simple definition of the future tense as *what will* be in the future. It moves beyond the future perfect tense of *that which will have* happened prior to a reference point in the future. It strives for the tense of possibility that grammarians refer to as the future real conditional or *that which will have* had to *happen.*
>
> (Campt, 2017, 34. Author's emphasis).

Dreaming a decolonized social work is not frivolous. It acknowledges the need for resilient, loving resistance and struggle to achieve a future that is beyond the oppressive structures of our current reality. And to reach that alternative reality, after the crisis of the COVID-19 pandemic and beyond, we must be able to dream beyond the limits of the coloniality of our current social work frameworks that often look to reform our colonized systems but not to fundamentally alter them.

Coloniality robs us of connecting with the true histories and wisdom of our ancestors. It limits our ability to understand and heal our trauma by erasing memory. In writing this book, we have been influenced by many outside of the field of social work, especially by young people, elders, artists, storytellers, knowledge keepers, fellow creatures, and Mother Earth. Their stories offer a different reckoning of how people who have been wounded and traumatized by the recurring narratives and brutal domination of empire, genocide, climate crisis, and the dividing lines of race, gender, and ability have nonetheless shown great strength and resilience to hope and thrive. To envision healing and lived experiences not based on exploitation, oppression, and greed, we must disrupt the narrow and familiar approaches upon which our structures and systems rely.

We offer this slim volume in recognition of the deeply compassionate social workers around the globe who strive every day to act in solidarity with distressed communities and individuals despite the limitations of working in agencies that use colonizing practices. Social workers sit with and bear witness to the pain and suffering of the most fragile in our communities, often with few tools to alleviate the hardship faced by their clients. Social workers are currently in the frontline of supporting people across the globe during the COVID-19 pandemic and will continue to be there long after the virus is controlled but the social consequences of the crisis remain.

We also write in recognition of the complexity of diverse communities and activists who have valiantly fought against unjust social systems and achieved real structural change. We are inspired by the daily struggle that so many sustain against settler colonialism in its manifold dimensions. We recognize the strength of social movements that have held many in power accountable and have pushed us forward in the struggle against coloniality, often at significant personal cost and despite huge barriers. We have been heartened by the fact that community-run mutual aid during the COVID-19 across the globe has been a significant support for people in need of food assistance, mental support, and myriad other needs.

We stand at a crossroads on the verge of climate catastrophe in the post-COVID-19 era: Do we continue down the road of settler colonialism and extractive capitalism, or can we fundamentally change our path? Can a new way of imaging a decolonized futurity help move social work as a profession beyond the confines of the current system?

Our aim with this book has been to challenge ourselves as social workers and community activists to fundamentally decenter coloniality from our ways of being, knowing, and acting. Can we dream a decolonized social work? As Maryan Abdulkarim has said, "Well, if we can't dream it, we sure can't build towards it." Let us reorient, reconfigure, restore, and remember ways of healing that have served us for millennia in a decolonized future.

References

Campt, T. 2017. *Listening to Images*. Durham, NC: Duke University Press.

Phillips, R. 2016. *Black Quantum Futurism: Space-Time Collapse I: From the Congo to the Carolinas*. Philadelphia: Afro Futurist Affairs Books.

Roy, A. 2020. The Pandemic Is a Portal. *Financial Times*, 3 April. Accessed 23 May 2020 at www.ft.com/content/10d8f5e8-74eb-11ea-95fe-fcd274e920ca.

Discussion guide

We hope that this book will encourage conversations around decolonization, social work, and healing. Here we have listed some prompts and tasks that we hope will lead to broader and engaged conversations.

Chapter 1

Consider your own profession or activism. How do our Western ways of being, knowing, and acting inform your practice? How do the processes and structures of settler colonialism inhibit the values, customs, and knowledge of people of color, diverse abilities, sexualities, genders, and other fragile and vulnerable groups in your practice or activism?

Chapter 2

What are some of the myriad ways colonialism continues to have an impact on us collectively and individually through historical trauma? How can we emerge from the shadow of historical trauma and use the power of memory begin to create another world?

Chapter 3

Confronting imperial professionalism is difficult, challenging, and scary because it is so embedded in the settler colonial structures of our society. How can we find ways to resist and reimagine other pathways to integrative healing?

Chapter 4

How does water have an impact on our well-being? How could activists and social workers integrate water at the center of their practice? How could social workers and other human service professionals become involved with ensuring access to clean water and protecting the intrinsic rights of water? How can we decolonize human-centered social work with regard to water?

Tasks:

- How can you help people in your communities create or remember stories about the sacredness of water? Document some of the stories.
- Where does your water come from? What does it mean to decolonize the use of water in your local context?
- Should every social work program be a green program? What would it look like if social work went green?

Chapter 5

How does creative expression influence our well-being? How are art and music used to colonize our understanding of history and ourselves? How can social workers and activists engage with communities to help understand the impact of forces of colonization through creative expression as a form of expression and resistance?
Tasks:

- Consider the difference between colonized and decolonized music. What are some of the ways that music has been used as a force for repression or liberation? Explore specific examples.
- How does art in your locale reinforce colonization or decolonize? Create a decolonized performance or art piece with community.
- What would a gallery of art and liberation made by social workers with the community look and sound like?

Chapter 6

How does movement have an impact on our well-being? Should social workers become involved with ensuring access to healthy movement? How can we use movement and play in direct social work practice? How could we decolonize movement and play in our communities and in our practice?
Tasks:

- Monitor your movement with a pedometer or your smartphone for a week. Reflect on how much you move and how this affects your sense of well-being.
- When was the last time you played? What did it feel like? Organize a collective event and unpack how it felt with participants.
- Take a walk in your neighborhood with a community member. How do people move and play?

Chapter 7

How do quiet and contemplation have an impact on well-being? What could be ways to incorporate quiet and contemplation in decolonized social work practice?

Tasks:

- What kinds of experiences of quiet and noise do you have in the world? Does silence and quiet differ to you? What are they like?
- With a partner, spend thirty minutes in quiet. What does it feel like? Reflect on the experience.
- For a week, track your moments of quiet, being on social media, in the midst of noise. Keep a journal and write how you feel during those moments.

Chapter 8

Do fellow creatures have the same rights as humans, and should they be treated as our equals? How do fellow creatures have an impact on our well-being? Should systems and institutions be more open to the presence of fellow creatures? How can we decolonize human-centered social work with regard to fellow creatures while honoring our community members who may have fear or trauma with fellow creatures?
　Tasks:

- How have fellow creatures been central to healing that you have observed, whether your own, another person's, or in a community?
- Take a neighborhood walk: What is the relationship of your place to fellow creatures?
- Interview your elders: What do their fellow creatures mean to them?

Chapter 9

How do social work structures and practices contain an extractive logic? What can we do in our practice to promote the rights of Mother Earth and to educate our communities about the importance of life in balance – and of understanding climate catastrophe? How can we decolonize human-centered social work?
　Tasks:

- According to your culture, your belief system, or your upbringing, what relationship are you intended to have with Mother Earth?
- Interview someone from a different culture or belief system and ask about their relationship with Mother Earth. Reflect on your differences.
- How has our educational training inculcated the value of Mother Earth in us?

Chapter 10

Imagine decolonized social work in your community – what would it look like in the future? How could we imagine a different way of supporting well-being in our communities and families in harmony with Mother Earth? How do you dream a decolonized futurity?

Index

Printed in the United States
By Bookmasters